Reviews and Advances in
BIOMECHANICS

Reviews and Advances in
BIOMECHANICS

Editors

Tung-Wu Lu
National Taiwan University, Taiwan

John K-J. Li
Rutgers University, USA

Li-Shan Chou
Iowa State University, USA

World Scientific

NEW JERSEY · LONDON · SINGAPORE · BEIJING · SHANGHAI · TAIPEI · CHENNAI

Published by

World Scientific Publishing Co. Pte. Ltd.
5 Toh Tuck Link, Singapore 596224
USA office: 27 Warren Street, Suite 401-402, Hackensack, NJ 07601
UK office: 57 Shelton Street, Covent Garden, London WC2H 9HE

British Library Cataloguing-in-Publication Data
A catalogue record for this book is available from the British Library.

REVIEWS AND ADVANCES IN BIOMECHANICS

ISBN 978-981-98-0610-2 (hardcover)
ISBN 978-981-98-0611-9 (ebook for institutions)
ISBN 978-981-98-0612-6 (ebook for individuals)

For any available supplementary material, please visit
https://www.worldscientific.com/worldscibooks/10.1142/14125#t=suppl

Typeset by Stallion Press
Email: enquiries@stallionpress.com

Contents

Preface

In the ever-evolving field of biomechanics research, the quest to understand and improve human health hinges on a multifaceted approach. This book is a comprehensive exploration of various methodologies and advancements aimed at deepening our understanding of arterial mechanics, joint dynamics, and gait balance analysis. Each chapter delves into distinct yet interconnected areas of study, reflecting the complexity of the human body and the sophistication required to evaluate its biomechanical properties.

Chapter 1, "Role of Arterial Compliance in Assessing the Biomechanical Properties of Arteries in Systole and Diastole and in Hypertension," provides a detailed examination of arterial compliance — a crucial factor in understanding cardiovascular health. This chapter investigates how the mechanical behavior of arteries during different phases of the cardiac cycle can be indicative of hypertension and other cardiovascular conditions. The subsequent chapter, "Noninvasive Brachial Artery Mechanics and Endothelial Function," shifts focus to the brachial artery, exploring noninvasive techniques to assess both its mechanical properties and endothelial function. This noninvasive approach is essential for early detection and management of vascular diseases. In "Analysis and Interpretation of Primary and Derived Data Sets in Cardiology," we dive into the methods of analyzing and interpreting complex data sets within the realm of cardiology. This chapter equips researchers and clinicians with the tools needed to derive meaningful insights from raw data, which is critical for advancing diagnostic and therapeutic strategies.

The book then transitions to a broader biomechanical perspective with Chapter 4, "Mathematical Model to Study the Squeeze Film Characteristics of Diseased Human Synovial Knee Joint." Here, we explore the application of mathematical models to understand the mechanics of knee joints affected by disease. This chapter illustrates the intersection of mathematics and biomechanics in addressing joint health issues. Continuing with our focus on structural mechanics, Chapter 5, "A Scoping Review of Current Methods and Limitations for Modeling and Evaluating Ligamentous Structures," offers a thorough review of the existing methods for studying ligamentous structures. This chapter identifies current practices, limitations, and future directions in the modeling and evaluation of these critical components of the musculoskeletal system. Finally, "Assessment of Gait Balance Control Using Inertial Measurement Units — A Narrative Review" wraps up the book by examining the role of inertial measurement units in evaluating gait balance control. This narrative review highlights the advancements in wearable technology and its impact on understanding and improving gait stability.

Together, these chapters present a holistic view of modern research and methodologies in cardiovascular, synovial joint, and gait balance studies. The integration of these diverse topics underscores the importance of interdisciplinary approaches in addressing complex health challenges. It is our hope that this book will serve as a valuable resource for researchers, clinicians, and students alike, fostering a deeper appreciation of the intricate dynamics of the human body and encouraging continued innovation in this vital field.

Li-Shan Chou
Department of Kinesiology,
Iowa State University, Ames. IA USA

Tung-Wu Lu
Department of Biomedical Engineering,
National Taiwan University, Taipei, Taiwan

John K-J. Li
Department of Biomedical Engineering,
Rutgers - The State University of New Jersey, Piscataway, NJ USA

CHAPTER 1

Role of Arterial Compliance in Assessing the Biomechanical Properties of Arteries in Systole and Diastole and in Hypertension[a]

John K-J. Li[*,§], Peter L. M. Kerkhof[†] and Mehmet Kaya[‡]

[*]*Department of Biomedical Engineering,*
Rutgers University, 599 Taylor Road, Piscataway, NJ 08854, USA

[†]*Department of Radiology and Nuclear Medicine Amsterdam, Cardiovascular Sciences,*
VU University Medical Center Amsterdam, The Netherlands

[‡]*Department of Biomedical and Chemical Engineering and Sciences,*
Florida Institute of Technology, Melbourne, FL, 32901, USA
[§]*johnkjli@soe.rutgers.edu*

The biomechanical properties of arteries play a crucial role in governing the overall hemodynamic function of the circulatory system. The nonuniformity in elastic and geometric structures of the blood vessels adds on to the complexity in dealing with pulsatile natures of blood pressure and flow. Short-term or chronic changes in arterial wall properties subjecting to distending pressure and perfusing flow make quantification of arterial compliance especially important in its use in describing the overall arterial function. This paper will first review the methodologies of determining arterial compliance in systole, in diastole and varying throughout the entire cardiac cycle. The stroke volume-to-pulse pressure method, the linear Windkessel model-based approaches and the nonlinear pressure-dependent compliance model method to derive arterial compliance are presented. The clinical relevance and implications are highlighted accordingly, in particular, the consequences of hypertension and aging.

Keywords: Arterial compliance; vascular stiffness; Windkessel; pressure-dependent compliance; aging; hypertension.

1. Introduction

The pulsatile nature of blood flow in the arterial system is manifested by the ejection of blood flow from the pumping heart. To receive the large amount of

---

[§]Corresponding author.
[a]This article was previously published in *World Scientific Annual Review of Biomechanics*. Vol: 1, (2023) 2330001 (21 pages).

blood ejected with each heartbeat, or stroke volume (SV), the connecting aorta must necessarily be compliant and readily distensible. The systolic pressure developed by the left ventricle (LV) that is transmitted through the aortic valve must exceed the pressure in the aorta (AoP) for ejection to occur. This pressure gradient becomes important in governing the flow. The resulting distending pressure exerted on the aorta is dependent on its wall properties. Thus, the interplay of pulsatile pressure (P), flow (Q) and volume (V) is intertwined. In fact, changes in P, Q and V are intimately dependent on the biomechanical properties of the arterial wall throughout the vascular tree. For this reason, transmission of such pressure and flow waveforms is modified as they travel to the periphery and to organ vascular beds.

Increased mean pressure increases vascular resistance. Increased pulse pressure (PP) is associated with increased vascular stiffness and decreased arterial compliance. The combination of increased mean pressure and pulse pressure thus precipitates to a further elevated blood pressure, a well-recognized predecessor to hypertension (Li, 2000a).

With increased blood pressure, the vessel distends to a larger diameter, but the proportional change in diameter with respect to its mean value, or radial strain, is greatly reduced. Vascular changes in hypertension differ among large and small arteries, arterioles and endothelial function. Vascular growth and hypertrophy associated with hypertension have also been frequently observed (e.g. Drzewiecki *et al.* 1997).

This paper will first review the methodologies of determining arterial compliance in systole, in diastole and throughout the entire cardiac cycle. The clinical relevance will be addressed, specifically how aging affects arterial compliance and how hypertension modifies blood vessels and precipitates changes in arterial compliance.

2. Arterial Compliance and Arterial Properties

2.1. *Definition of arterial compliance*

The general definition of arterial compliance (C) is the ratio of an incremental change in volume due to an incremental change in distending pressure, i.e.

$$C = dV/dP. \tag{1}$$

This is defined by the inverse of the slope of the pressure–volume (P–V) curve shown in Fig. 1, with pressure plotted on the ordinate and volume on the abscissa. Thus, compliance is the inverse of stiffness.

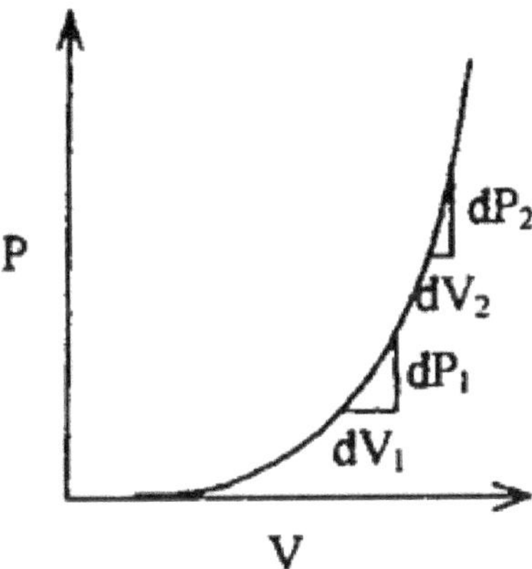

Fig. 1.   Arterial *P–V* diagram, defining compliance as the slope of the relation: $C = dV/dP$. It is clear that the slope change is steeper, resulting in compliance that decreases with increasing pressure $(dV_2/dP_2 < dV_1/dP_1)$.

For arteries, C represents the vessel volume displacement (dV) due to pulsatile flowing blood and the distending pulsatile pressure (dP). Compliance value varies in different arteries, depending on the magnitude of the pressure pulse and the ability to distend. Compliance can be expressed for a specific artery or its segment. Total compliance, such as defined by SV/PP, can also be quantified for the entire arterial system, as commonly done in clinical situations.

Large arteries, such as the aorta, have greater displacement in volume subjecting to any given pulse pressure and correspondingly contribute to more of the total arterial system compliance. This makes large artery compliance a significant parameter for clinical monitoring, particularly that of the proximal aorta.

The pressure–volume curves of arteries have been found to be curvilinear as seen in Fig. 1. The slope change along the *P–V* curve is steeper at higher pressures, signifying increased arterial stiffness or decreased compliance and distensibility. In other words, arteries stiffen when pressurized, associated with increased shear stress. This physiological phenomenon has been experimentally and clinically observed (e.g. Cox, 1975; Thubrikar and Robicsek, 1995). The increased stiffness is related to the structure of the arterial wall. This implies that the compliance–pressure relation is not a constant one. The declining arterial compliance with increasing pressure has been observed in the central aorta and in individual arteries (Li, 2000a, 2018b). This inverse exponential relation between compliance and pressure for the arterial system is clearly shown in Fig. 2.

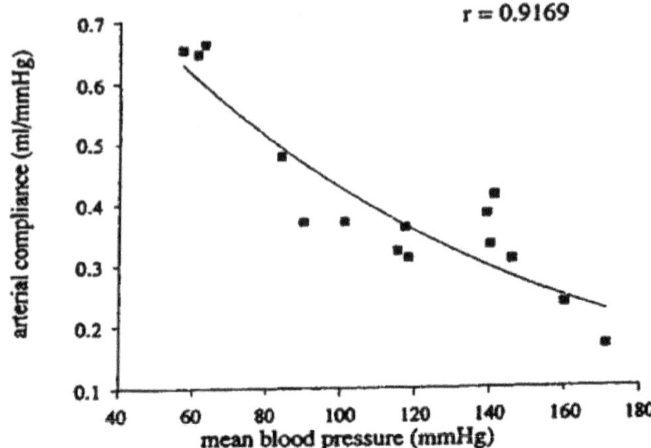

Fig. 2.   Experimentally obtained arterial compliance plotted against mean blood pressure reflecting the pressure–volume relation. The relationship is nonlinear, implying that at higher distending pressures the intraluminal volume change is smaller, resulting in a lower compliance. The decrease in arterial compliance with increasing blood pressure follows a negative exponential function.

2.2. Elastic and viscoelastic properties of blood vessels

To deal with arterial compliance, we must know the composite physical behavior of the arterial wall. A simplistic cross-sectional view (Fig. 3) reveals the tunica intima, which is the innermost layer consisting of a thin layer (0.5–1 μm) of endothelial cells, connective tissue and basement membrane. The middle layer is the thick tunica media, separated from the intima by a prominent layer of elastic tissue, the internal lamina. The media contains elastin, smooth muscle cells and collagen fibers. The outermost layer is the adventitia which is made up mostly of stiff fibrous collagen. The differences in the wall compositions separate arteries into large elastic arteries, such as the aorta, and smaller muscular arteries, such as the femoral and radial arteries.

Elastic laminae are concentrically distributed in the media and attached by smooth muscle cells and connective tissue. Longitudinally, one observes that the number of elastic laminae decreases with increasing distance from the aorta, but the amount of smooth muscle increases and the relative wall thickness increases. As a result, the wall-thickness-to-radius ratio, or h/r, is increased. The net increase in vascular stiffness accounts for the increase in pulse wave velocity (PWV) toward the periphery, as seen from the Moens–Korteweg formula relating propagating speed of the arterial pulse to the conduit arterial elasticity and geometry (Li, 1987, 2004). The mechanical behavior of small peripheral arteries can be largely

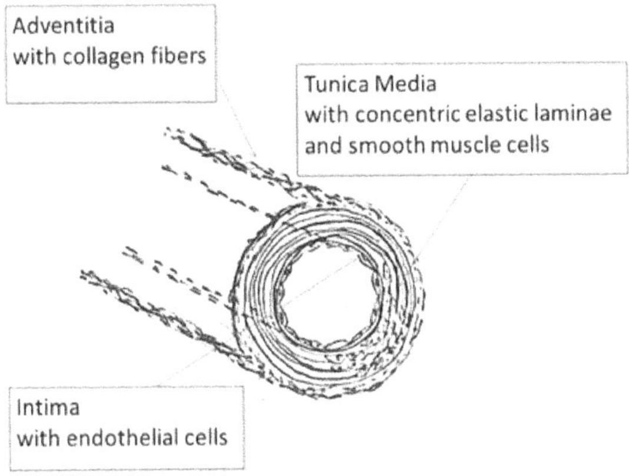

Fig. 3.   Sketch of the cross-sections of the artery reveals three distinctive layers: the thin innermost tunica intima, the thick distensible tunica media and the stiff outermost adventitia.

influenced by the behavior of the smooth muscle, particularly by the degree of its activation.

The extracellular matrix components, or those of elastin and collagen, govern the passive mechanical properties of the large and small arteries. There have been numerous studies in experimental animals and in humans (e.g. Wagenseil and Mecham, 2012; Villard *et al.*, 2014). The contribution of vascular smooth muscle (VSM) to overall arterial wall properties and hemodynamic function has also been continually investigated (e.g. Somlyo and Somlyo, 1968; van Loo *et al.*, 2022).

2.3. *Vascular stiffness and arterial wall stress–strain relations*

The stiffness of an artery is inversely related to its compliance. Stiffness is traditionally expressed in terms of Young's modulus of elasticity, which gives a simple description of the elastic properties of the arterial wall. Young's modulus of elasticity (E) is defined by the ratio of tensile stress (σ_t) to tensile strain (ε_t). When the relationship between stress and strain is a linear one, then the material is said to be Hookean, or simply, it obeys Hooke's law of elasticity. This normally applies to a purely elastic material. It is only valid for application to a cylindrical blood vessel when the radial and longitudinal deformations are small compared to the respective lumen diameter or length of the arterial segment.

It has been recognized that the arterial wall is anisotropic (e.g. Noordergraaf, 1969; Weizsacker and Pascal, 1982) consisting of various components exhibiting an intertwined elastic behavior, as we discussed above. However, assumption of isotropy is common to allow simpler clinical quantitative descriptions of the mechanical behavior of the arterial wall properties and eases mathematical computation. More detailed treatment of biomechanical properties of the viscoelastic arterial wall can be found, for instance, in Noordergraaf (1969); Fung (1997) and (Humphrey, 2013). Below, we provide the basic biomechanical elements that are clinically applicable.

Consider a cylindrical isotropic arterial segment with radius r, wall thickness h and segment length l, then the Young's modulus of elasticity in terms of tensile stress and tensile strain is

$$E = \frac{\sigma_t}{\varepsilon_t}. \tag{2}$$

Stress has the dimension of pressure, or force (F) per unit area (A),

$$\sigma_t = \frac{F}{A} = P, \tag{3}$$

where P is the pressure.

Strain in the longitudinal direction, or along the length of the blood vessel, is expressed as the ratio of extension per unit length, or the ratio of the amount stretched longitudinally, to the length of the original vessel segment,

$$\varepsilon_t = \frac{\Delta l}{l}. \tag{4}$$

Strain in the radial direction, or perpendicular to the vessel segment length, is the fraction of distention of the vessel lumen radius or diameter. It is given by

$$\varepsilon_r = \frac{\Delta r}{r}. \tag{5}$$

Poisson's ratio describes compressibility and is defined as the ratio of radial strain to longitudinal strain,

$$\sigma_n = \frac{\varepsilon_r}{\varepsilon_t} = \frac{\Delta r/r}{\Delta l/l}. \tag{6}$$

When $\sigma_n = 0.5$, the material is said to be incompressible. This means that when a cylindrical artery is stretched, its volume remains unchanged. Experimental measurements to obtain the Poisson's ratio for arteries have shown σ_n to be about 0.48, or close to 0.5. Arteries, therefore, can be considered to be close to being incompressible.

Clearly, a purely elastic material differs from a viscoelastic material, such as an artery. The former depends only on strain, while the latter also depends on the rate of change of strain, or strain rate $(d\varepsilon/dt)$. The artery as a viscoelastic material exhibits stress-relaxation, creep and hysteresis phenomena (Li, 2004).

Hysteresis develops when the vessel is subjected to sinusoidal or cyclic changes. If the artery is purely elastic, there will be no phase shift between the applied pressure and the resulting change in diameter. That is, the diameter waveform will resemble pressure waveform exactly. The viscoelastic behavior of the artery leads to phase shifts in its pressure–diameter relation. Thus a hysteresis loop is observed. In other words, energy is dissipated due to viscous losses in stretching the artery and subsequently allowing it to return to its control value. If the artery were purely elastic, there would be no energy loss and the artery would return to its control value along the exact path as during stretching. This follows the curvilinear pressure–volume relation of arterial compliance we saw above.

Examples of experimentally measured pressure–diameter relations are shown in Fig. 4 for the pulmonary aorta. Since the pulmonary aorta is normally oval, there are two different diameters, namely, the major axis diameter and the minor axis diameter. When the major and minor axes diameters are plotted against pressure, the hysteresis loops are clearly seen. It is also clear that the pulmonary aorta is stiffer (less diameter distention with increasing pressure) along the major axis than the minor axis. In small muscular arteries, such as the femoral artery, the viscous modulus is larger and the phase shift becomes more pronounced.

Changes in arterial wall thickness, h, often accompany radial changes (Li, 2004; Noordergraaf, 2011). When h is taken into account, the relative volume (V)

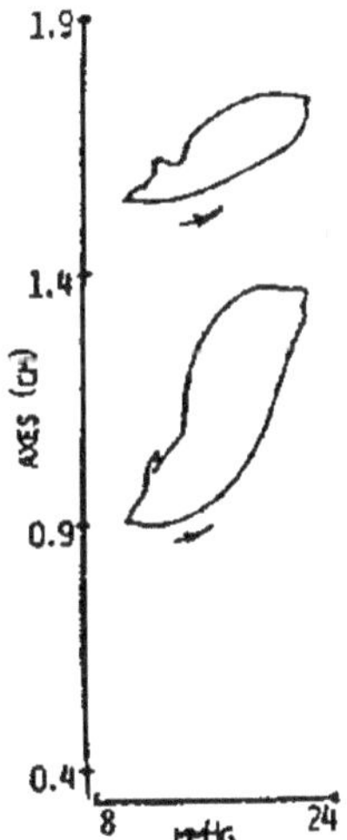

Fig. 4.   Pressure–diameter relation of the main pulmonary artery showing hysteresis loops. Top tracing: major axis. Bottom tracing: minor axis. The difference in hysteresis loops is due to the noncylindrical oval cross-sectional shape of the main pulmonary artery.

distensibility of the artery is given by

$$\frac{dV}{VdP} = \frac{3rV}{2hE}.$$ (7)

The magnitude of the ratio h/r separates arteries into "thin-walled" and "thick-walled" vessels. Thus, an increase in wall thickness or lumen radius alone can impact the overall distensibility of the artery. The consequence of this has been found to be particularly important in the clinical condition of vascular hypertrophy. Thickening of the arterial wall is largely due to the remodeling in the tunica media.

Laplace's law can be useful in quantifying the tension (T) exerted on the arterial wall due to intraluminal pulsatile blood pressure distention. In the case of blood vessels, there are two radii of curvature. In the radial direction, Laplace's law for a thin-walled ($h/r \leq 1/10$) artery is given as

$$T = p \cdot r,$$ (8)

where p is the transmural pressure. For a thick-walled artery, we have

$$\sigma_t = \frac{pr}{h}.$$ (9)

In hypertension, however, tension can be normalized by increasing the arterial wall thickness. Such chronic increase often leads to observed vascular hypertrophy (Li, 1986, 1996, 2000b).

Collagen is the stiffest wall component, with an elastic modulus of 10^8–10^9 dyn/cm^2. This is some two orders of magnitude greater than those of elastin [$(1-6) \times 10^6$ dyn/cm^2] and smooth muscle [$(0.1-2.5) \times 10^6$ dyn/cm^2]. Elastin is relatively extensible, but is not a purely Hookean material. Collagen on the other hand is relatively inextensible, because of its high elastic stiffness. Vascular smooth muscle can appreciably alter its elastic stiffness upon activation. The overall composite of the arterial wall components operates in such a manner that at low pressures, elastin dominates the composite behavior. At high pressures, collagen becomes more dominant. As a result, arterial compliance can alter considerably during different pathological conditions due to the interplay of the ratio of collagen to elastin and the extent of VSM activation (e.g. Atlas and Li, 2009; Craim *et al.*, 2012).

The characteristics of a viscoelastic biological material such as the arterial wall concern stress-relaxation, creep phenomenon and hysteresis which is associated with dissipative energy loss. If a strip of artery is subjected to a step change in length, it will result in an initial increase in stress, and then a decay to a lower value. This is known as stress-relaxation. There is a finite amount of time the vessel takes to relax. This is described by a time constant, which differs in different arteries. When an artery is subjected to a stepwise change in stress, its length will gradually increase to a constant value. This is the so-called "creep phenomenon". As with stress-relaxation, the increase in length or diameter also takes a finite amount of time and is again described by a time constant. These properties allow arteries to respond to rapid transient changes in transmural blood pressures.

2.4. *Pressure–strain elastic modulus and dynamic elastic modulus*

2.4.1. *Pressure–strain elastic modulus*

From the fractional change in pulsatile diameter, $\Delta D/D$, and the pulsatile change in pressure from systole to diastole, or pulse pressure, the difference between systolic (P_s) and diastolic (P_d) pressures, i.e. $\Delta P = P_s - P_d$, the pressure–strain elastic modulus can be obtained, viz.

$$Ep = \frac{\Delta P}{(\Delta D/D)}.\tag{10}$$

Thus, simultaneous recordings of pressure–diameter relations allow E_p to be readily computed, such as that shown in Fig. 5 from ultrasonic dimension gages-recorded aortic diameter and catheterization-recorded aortic pressure. E_p is more commonly obtained noninvasively in the clinical setting with *M*-mode

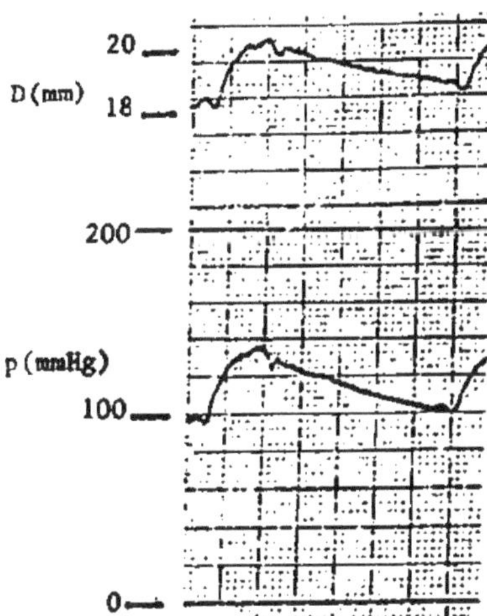

Fig. 5.   Ultrasonic dimension gages-recorded diameter of the dog aorta, together with aortic blood pressure, showing how pressure–strain elastic modulus, E_p, can be computed from the pressure–diameter relation: $E_p = \Delta P/(\Delta D/D)$, where $\Delta P = \mathrm{PP}$.

echocardiography for diameter measurement and brachial artery cuff for pulse pressure estimation.

2.4.2. *Dynamic elastic modulus*

The static modulus of elasticity differs from the dynamic elastic value. Measurement of dynamic elasticity (E_{dyn}) has gained considerable attention, mainly because of its applicability to pulsatile conditions. The approach employs the measurement of pressure–diameter relations, and the subsequent calculations of the incremental elastic modulus (E_{inc}) which is complex (E_c):

$$E_{inc} = E_{dyn} + \eta\omega. \tag{11}$$

When an elastic modulus is complex, it implies frequency-dependence. The in-phase component defines the dynamic elastic modulus,

$$E_{dyn} = |E_c|\cos\phi, \tag{12}$$

and the viscous modulus is defined by

$$\eta\omega = |E_c|\sin\phi, \tag{13}$$

where ϕ is the phase lag, generally between pressure (P) and diameter (D). In the case that pressure leads diameter, or that the diameter distention delays after the arrival of the pressure pulse, ϕ is positive. When E_{dyn} is plotted as a function of frequency for the thoracic aorta, abdominal aorta, femoral and carotid arteries, E_{dyn} is essentially unchanged above 2 Hz.

Experimental results show that the viscous modulus is small compared with the elastic modulus (Li *et al.*, 1981; Li, 1987; Westerhof and Noordergraaf, 1970). It is of the order of 10%. Although Maxwell and Voigt models have been used to describe arterial viscoelasticity, they have their shortcomings. In a Maxwell model, creep is unbounded, whereas in a Voigt model, stress-relaxation is unbounded (Li, 2018a).

3. Compliance Determined in Systole as Defined by Stoke Volume to Pulse Pressure or $C = SV/PP$

3.1. *Arterial compliance obtained during ventricular systole*

With each ventricular systole, the amount of blood ejected is the stroke volume. The most common estimation of arterial compliance is thus based on its fundamental definition $C = dV/dP$, with change in volume during the heart beat as

$SV = dV$ and change in pressure dP from the difference of arterial systolic pressure (P_s) and diastolic pressure (P_d), or simply the pulse pressure, given that $PP = P_s - P_d$.

While PP is relatively easier to account for, arterial volume is difficult to measure in practice. Thus, SV has been used as a surrogate of a measure of total arterial volume, hence

$$C_v = SV/PP. \tag{14}$$

Note here that stroke volume is determined in systole during ventricular ejection, whereas pulse pressure is determined in the entire cardiac cycle.

The inverse relation of pulse pressure to arterial compliance has been well documented. Experimental studies have shown that the majority ($\sim$60%) (e.g. Stergiopulos *et al.* 1999) of the total arterial system compliance resides in the proximal aorta.

3.2. *Clinical measurement of stroke volume-to-pulse pressure ratio*

Noninvasively, in humans, our group was one of the first to demonstrate the combined use of ultrasound imaging for change in volume and tonometer pulse pressure for the SV/PP arterial compliance determination (e.g. Iantorno and Li, 1988). This method was also utilized by Haluska *et al.* (2010) in assessing arterial compliance as an independent predictor of cardiovascular events. More recently, Bahlmann *et al.* (2019) utilized Doppler echocardiograph and brachial blood pressure to give SV/PP found in patients with aortic valve stenosis that low systemic arterial compliance is associated with increased morbility and mortality. This followed similar findings in an earlier study by our group in humans (Ilercil *et al.*, 1995). We have been able to predict the consequence of pressure-induced hypertrophy due to a double-loaded ventricle, i.e. hypertension plus aortic valve stenosis (Li *et al.*, 1997).

Invasively, the SV/PP approach was followed by Chemla *et al.* (1998) in clinical settings during catheterization for aortic pulse pressure measurement and thermodilution to provide cardiac output. Similarly, Fagard *et al.* (2001) utilized catheterization and Fick's dilution cardiac output method to infer PP/SV ratio (inverse of SV/PP) as a predictor of cardiovascular events and mortality in hypertensives. de Simone *et al.* (1999) showed that the survival rate for patients with reduced SV/PP ratio is considerably less than those with higher SV/PP ratio, when age and left ventricular mass are taken into account.

For the right heart, reduced pulmonary arterial compliance was a limiting factor in exercise capacity in patients after pulmonary endarterectomy

(Ghio *et al.*, 2014). It should be noted here that pulmonary arterial compliance is normally considerably larger than the total systemic arterial compliance.

4. Compliance Determined in Diastole based on the Windkessel Model

4.1. *Relating arterial wall properties to pulsatile pressure and flow*

The storage properties of blood in large arteries and their distensibility are important transforming the intermittent outflow of the heart to steady outflow to the peripheral vessels. Thus, the large overall "compliance" of these arteries protects the stiff peripheral vessels of organ vascular beds from the large swings in pulsatile pressure. This resulted in the well-known lumped Windkessel model of the arterial system, seen in Fig. 6.

4.2. *Determining arterial compliance in diastole based on the Windkessel model*

Considering the Windkessel model, the amount of blood flow, Q_s, stored during each LV contraction is the difference between inflow, Q_i, to the large arteries and the outflow, Q_o, to the small peripheral vessel (Fig. 6),

$$Q_s = Q_i - Q_o. \tag{15}$$

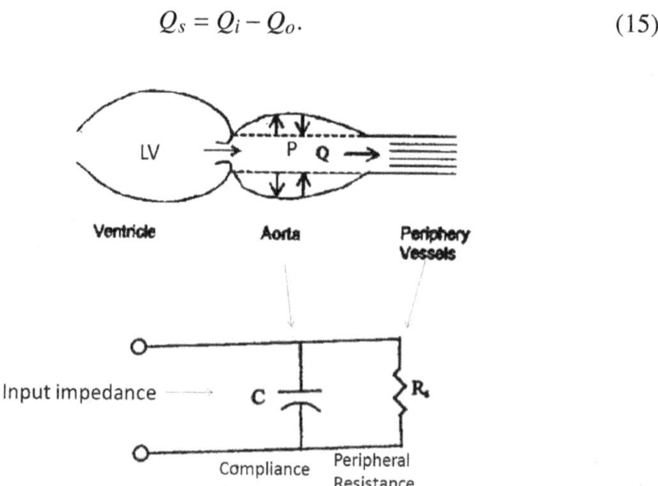

Fig. 6.   Illustration of the left ventricle and the connecting arterial circulation based on the two-element Windkessel model. The ventricle ejects into a compliant chamber representing the aorta, blood flow is stored in systole (solid line) and on diastolic elastic recoil (dotted line) stiff peripheral vessels are perfused. Compliance is represented by an energy-storing capacitor and the peripheral resistance by an energy-dissipating resistor.

The amount of outflow is equivalent to the pressure drop from the arterial side (P) to the venous side (P_v) due to the peripheral resistance, R_s,

$$Q_o = (P - P_v)/R_s. \tag{16}$$

Since P_v is small, and with the total inflow $Q = Q_i$, we obtain

$$R_s = \bar{P}/\bar{Q}, \tag{17}$$

or the ratio of mean arterial pressure to mean arterial flow. Again, compliance is

$$C = dV/dP. \tag{18}$$

Blood flow stored, due to arterial compliance, is related to the rate of change in pressure distending the artery,

$$Q_s = CdP/dt. \tag{19}$$

Substituting (16) and (19) into (15), then we have

$$Q(t) = CdP/dt + P/R_s. \tag{20}$$

That is, the total arterial inflow is the sum of the flow stored in the aorta and the flow going into the periphery.

In diastole, aortic flow equals zero after aortic valve closure, so we have

$$0 = CdP/dt + P/R_s \tag{21}$$

or

$$dP/P = -dt/R_sC. \tag{22}$$

On integration, we have

$$P_d = P_{es}e^{-td/\tau}. \tag{23}$$

Thus, during the diastolic period (t_d), the rate of diastolic aortic pressure decay from end-systolic pressure (P_{es}) to diastolic pressure (P_d), as shown in Fig. 7, is dependent on both the compliance of the arterial system and the total peripheral resistance, as characterized by a time constant,

$$\tau = R_sC, \tag{24}$$

or in terms of the measured aortic pressure,

$$\tau = \frac{t_d}{\ln \frac{P_{es}}{P_d}} \tag{25}$$

and

$$C = \frac{t_d}{R_s \ln \frac{P_{es}}{P_d}}. \tag{26}$$

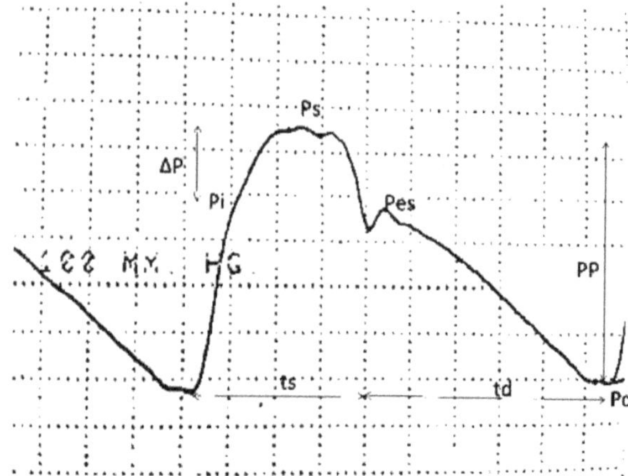

Fig. 7.   Illustration of the measured aortic pressure pulse waveform for defining the systolic pressure P_s, diastolic pressure P_d, end-systolic pressure P_{es}, pulse pressure $PP = P_s - P_d$, inflection pressure P_i and the augmented systolic pressure $\Delta P = P_s - P_i$.

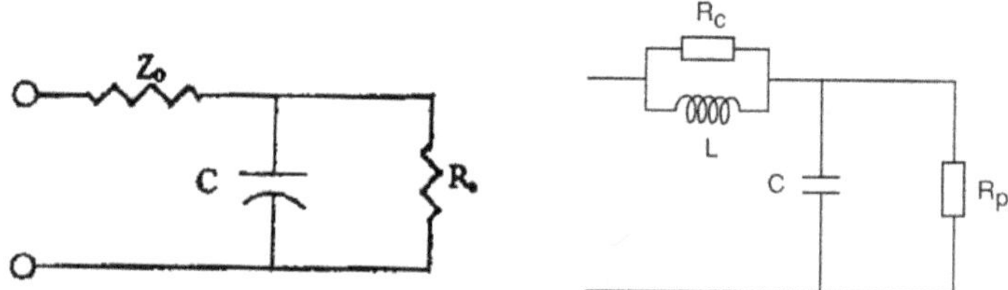

Fig. 8.   The three-element Windkessel model with Z_o representing the characteristic impedance of the proximal aorta (left). Viscous property inclusion results in an additional resistive element in parallel with the compliance element. The four-element model of the arterial system with inertia represented by an inductance (right).

The three-element Windkessel model (Fig. 8) of the arterial system is now more widely used, incorporating a characteristic impedance of the proximal aorta or Z_o, but compliance is still determined from the exponential diastolic aortic pressure decay ($\tau = R_sC$), as with the four-element model ($\tau = R_pC$).

4.3. *Pulse contour methods to determine arterial compliance*

A variation to the Windkessel model is the use of aortic pressure pulse contour for the determination of arterial compliance, as shown by Goldwyn and Watt (1967) and Watt and Burrus (1976). This was followed by the separation of large artery compliance and small artery compliance approaches calculated from the diastolic pressure decays using a third-order four-element modified Windkessel model (e.g. McVeigh *et al.* 1999; Syeda *et al.* 2003). Comparison of different approaches has also been investigated (e.g. Resnick *et al.*, 2000; Boutouyrie, 2008; Sakuragi and Abhayaratna, 2010; Haluska *et al.*, 2010).

Laskey *et al.* (1990) estimated the total systemic arterial compliance in humans. Marcus *et al.* (1994) provided a noninvasive approach using tonometer for subclavian arterial pressure and echocardiographic Doppler to evaluate arterial compliance based on the Windkessel two- and three-element models and found the latter had a somewhat smaller compliance values.

The Windkessel model compliance is determined in diastole only. Some investigators have utilized both the systolic and diastolic information contained in the pressure waveform and used the area method (e.g. Liu *et al.* 1986) for calculating the total arterial compliance,

$$C = \frac{\text{DPTI/SV}}{(\text{SPTI} + \text{DPTI}) \cdot \text{PP}}, \tag{27}$$

where SPTI and DPTI are systolic and diastolic time integrals, respectively.

5. Continuous Compliance Variation Throughout the Cardiac Cycle as Determined from Nonlinear Arterial Compliance Model

5.1. *Instantaneous or pressure-dependent arterial compliance observations*

The pressure-dependence of arterial compliance has been well recognized and is commonly referred from experimental observations that arteries stiffen when pressurized. The decreased compliance with increasing blood pressure is more pronounced in large vessels, such as the aorta. This phenomenon has also been observed in other arteries in experimental animals (e.g. Cox, 1975) and in humans. This increased stiffness is associated with changes in the structural component properties of the arterial walls. Thus, the compliance–pressure relation is not a constant one. This Windkessel model formulated above assumes that the compliance of the arterial system remains constant throughout the cardiac cycle. Hence, compliance in systole and in diastole is assumed to be the same, despite continuously varying blood pressure amplitudes. We have shown that pulse pressure is a significant determinant of arterial compliance, even within a single cardiac cycle (Li *et al.*, 1994).

It has been found that elastic modulus is a nonlinear function of pressure. The pressure-dependence of the mechanical properties of arteries has been reported by several investigators (e.g. Cox, 1975; Li and Zhu, 1994; Drzewiecki *et al.*, 1997;

Wells *et al.*, 1998). With increasing positive transmural pressure, arterial vessel diameter is distended (Weizsacker and Pascal, 1982) while the corresponding compliance however declines.

5.2. *Nonlinear aspects and pressure-dependent arterial compliance*

Our group was the first to demonstrate that continuous changes in total arterial system compliance can be quantified (Li *et al.*, 1990). A nonlinear model of the arterial system incorporating a pressure-dependent compliance element $[C(P)]$ is shown below. The model consists of the characteristic impedance of the proximal aorta (Z_o), the peripheral resistance (R_s) and $C(P)$. The compliance is exponentially related to pressure and is expressed as

$$C(P) = a \cdot e^{b(P(t))}, \tag{28}$$

where a and b are constants. The exponent b is normally negative. Thus, an inverse relationship is established between arterial compliance and blood pressure; with increasing blood pressure the arterial compliance decreases. Arterial compliance, either of a single vessel or of the whole arterial system, has been shown to be dependent on the level of blood pressure in an inverse exponential relation (Li *et al.*, 1990; Matonick and Li, 2001; Kaya *et al.*, 2018).

Figure 9 shows that the flow through the compliance branch of the nonlinear model is given by

$$Q_c(t) = Q(t) - P(t)/R_s, \tag{29}$$

where $P(t)$ and $Q(t)$ are the pressure and flow through the compliance branch, respectively. This flow can also be expressed as

$$Q_c(t) = C(P) \cdot dP(t)/dt. \tag{30}$$

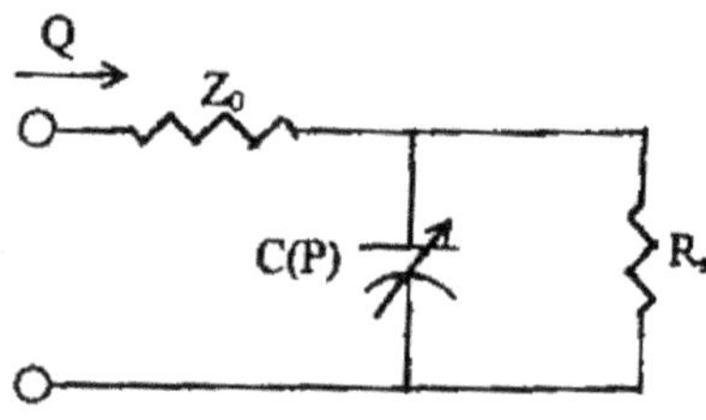

Fig. 9.   Nonlinear arterial system model according to Li *et al.* (1990), incorporating a pressure-dependent compliance. Z_o is the characteristic impedance of the ascending aorta, R_s is the total peripheral resistance, $C(P)$ is the pressure-dependent compliance, represented by a variable capacitor, and Q is aortic flow.

Equating these two equations thus results in

$$dP/dt = (Q(t) - P(t)/R_s)/C(P). \tag{31}$$

This equation defines the dynamic relationship between pressure and flow for a nonlinear compliance element. Numerical methods can be employed to solve this equation.

Using difference representations, we have

$$\Delta t = t_{i+1} - t_i = dt, \tag{32}$$

where Δt is the sampling interval, taken as 10 ms. The nonlinear model is then reduced to the following expression:

$$P(t_{i+1}) = P(t_i) + \Delta t \cdot (Q(t_i) - P(t_i)/R_s)/C(P). \tag{33}$$

With the measured aortic flow as the input, a numerical procedure can be programmed to solve $P(t_i)$, $C(P)$ and the aortic pressure

$$P_a(t_i) = Q(t_i) \cdot Z_o + P(t_i). \tag{34}$$

The linear three-element model predicted the measured aortic pressure with less accuracy, although the gross features are evident. The nonlinear model-based arterial compliance plotted as a function of pressure for a complete cardiac cycle with a normal blood pressure level is shown in Fig. 10. Compliance maintains a value close to its maximum to facilitate early rapid ventricular ejection. Arterial system compliance reaches its minimum at the end of the ejection. For the

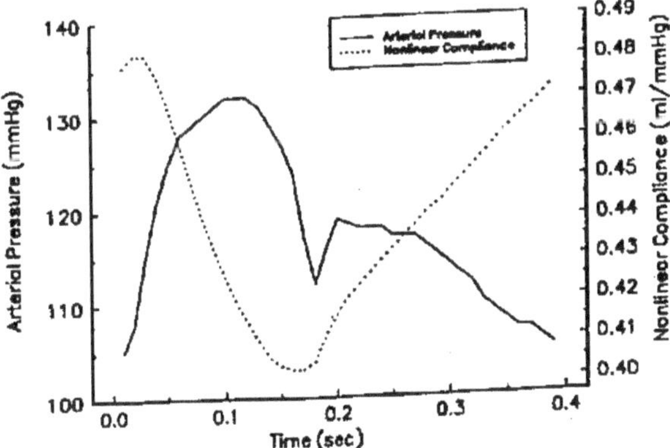

Fig. 10.   Nonlinear pressure-dependent characteristics of arterial compliance as a function of time plotted for a complete cardiac cycle. Arterial compliance increases initially at the beginning of ejection and declines with increasing pressure. It reaches a minimum at about end-systole and increases steadily thence toward the end of diastole.

diastolic period, when aortic flow is zero, compliance increases following an exponential relation with declining pressure. Its value increases throughout the diastole toward maximum, readying for the following ventricular ejection (Li, 2000a; Matonick and Li, 2001; Kaya *et al.*, 2018).

Arterial compliance and blood pressure bear a close relation. As such, the continuously varying compliance–pressure loop actually represents a logical new approach to describing blood vessel properties (Li, 1998; Kaya *et al.*, 2018). It allows visualization of vessel lumen geometry changes in relation to mechanical property alteration throughout the cardiac cycle (Li, 1998). This can be well illustrated when the compliance–pressure loops for control, methoxamine-induced hypertension and vasodilation-induced profound vasodilation are plotted on a single graph as illustrated in Fig. 11. Here, the compliance change over the entire range of blood pressures (50–200 mmHg) is clearly seen, i.e. compliance decreases with increasing pressure. More importantly, the range of compliance variation within a cardiac cycle is significantly reduced in hypertension, despite large distending pressure, indicating increased vascular stiffness. In contrast, vasodilation with nitroprusside is associated with a large compliance–pressure loop area, accompanied by significantly increased compliance.

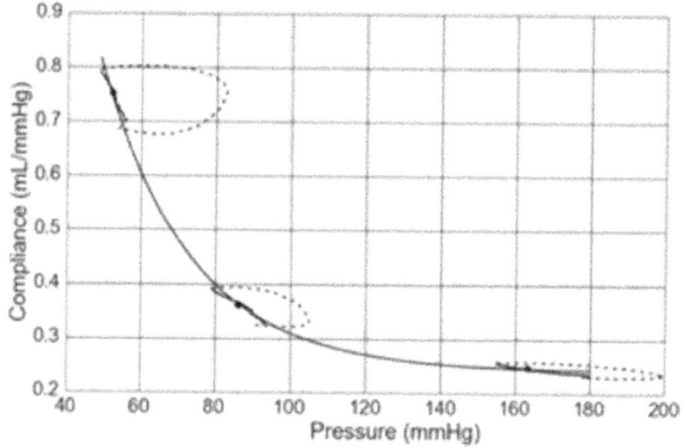

Fig. 11.   Compliance versus pressure (solid line) and compliance–pressure loops (dotted lines) plotted for the control (middle), methoxamine-induced hypertension (right) and nitroprusside-induced vasodilation (left) cases. Note that the overall compliance decreases with increasing pressure and that the loop area is compressed in hypertension and enlarged with vasodilator.

6. Arterial Compliance in Aging and Hypertension

6.1. *Definition of hypertension*

There are several forms of hypertension. The most common form is known as essential hypertension whose origins are still unclear. In this review, focus will be on the hemodynamic aspects of hypertension. Brachial artery cuff method has become the norm for defining blood pressure levels. Systolic/diastolic pressure of 120/80 mmHg has been defined as normal and 130/90 mmHg is classified as hypertensive. It should be noted here that brachial arterial systolic pressure is normally greater and diastolic pressure smaller than the central aortic pressure. This is reflected in the Strong Heart Study where central pressure has been shown to be more strongly related to vascular disease and outcome than does brachial pressure (Roman *et al.*, 2007).

6.2. *Arterial compliance and peripheral resistance alterations in hypertension*

Arterial compliance and peripheral vascular resistance comprise the major components of the ventricular load. It has been shown that reduced arterial compliance and/or increased peripheral resistance impedes ventricular ejection. Increased arterial pressure has been shown to reduce myocardial shortening (Li, 2000a). Concentric left ventricular hypertrophy (LVH) has been found to be associated with increased carotid arterial wall thickness, cross-sectional area and elastic modulus (Ilercil *et al.*, 1995) when simultaneous noninvasive recordings of the carotid pulse and vessel diameter by *M*-mode ultrasound echocardiograph were performed. In general, chronic hypertension promotes concentric LVH.

In vascular hypertrophy and hypertension, biomechanical changes are observed with selective thickening in tunica media accompanied by an increase in collagen and a decrease in elastin, and/or a change in the level of smooth muscle activation. However, these observed changes are not uniform throughout the arterial wall, i.e. anisotropic. Hypertension directly reflects the increased tension on the blood vessel wall.

Arterial hypertension has been associated with an increased peripheral resistance. The concurrent reduction in arterial compliance has also been reported (e.g. Berger and Li, 1990). Alterations in compliance and resistance reflect underlying changes in the biomechanical properties of the vessel walls and the state of the perfused vascular beds (Li, 1987, 2000a; Armentano *et al.*, 1991). Successful antihypertensive therapy must be able to normalize both vascular resistance and compliance in order to have any long-term impact. This may rely on adequate vascular remodeling of the biomechanical properties.

The compliance–pressure curve has been given by some investigators for individual arteries, such as the human radial and brachial arteries (e.g. Perret *et al.* 1991). The pressure–strain elastic modulus is more popular because of its ease of measurements in clinical situations in assessing the arterial compliance or distensibility.

The effects on blood pressure due to changes in arterial compliance and peripheral resistance are quite well known. An increase in R_s results in an increased mean pressure, and if C is unchanged, the systolic and diastolic pressures would both increase. Changing C should have no effect on the mean pressure, if the flow waveform remains unchanged. A decrease in C would result in an increased systolic pressure and a decreased diastolic pressure. Specifically, the effect of decreasing C and increasing R_s would result in a combined and a larger increase in P_s than P_d. Changing C can alter the arrival of wave reflections and can significantly alter systolic blood pressure (Li *et al.*, 2010; Phan *et al.*, 2016).

6.3. *Aging and hypertension*

Iantorno and Li (1988) have investigated changes in total arterial compliance in three different types of hypertension. Arterial compliances calculated from the diastolic aortic pressure decay time constant (C_t) and the ratio of stroke volume to pulse pressure (C_v) were compared in four groups of subjects. These are normal (N) adults, isolated systolic hypertensives (ISH), diastolic hypertensives (DH) and hypertensives with both elevated systolic and diastolic blood pressures (SDH). All hypertensives are seen to have reduced total arterial system compliance when compared to normal individuals. The decrease is small in diastolic hypertensives, mostly due to lower pulse pressure and overall mean pressure. It is well recognized that with advance age, arterial compliance decreases. With age, elderly patients with ISH and SDH exhibit significantly greater reduction in arterial compliance (e.g. Berger and Li, 1990; van Bortel and Spek, 1998; Papaioannou *et al.*, 2014). In addition, it can be seen that either method of determining arterial compliance can differentiate the arterial compliance changes. It has been recognized that aging is associated with early arrival of reflected waves (e.g. Li *et al.* 2007; Phan *et al.* 2016) and this resulted in significantly reduced total arterial system compliance (Li, 2000b; Li *et al.*, 2007).

7. Arterial Compliance in Relation to Other Indices of Vascular Stiffness

Several other hemodynamic indices have been used to quantify arterial compliance indirectly, most commonly, pulse wave velocity (PWV). This is because PWV is the clinically accepted index of vascular stiffness and arterial compliance is the inverse of vascular stiffness discussed earlier. Vascular stiffness indices such as PWV, pulse wave reflection (WR) and augmentation index (Aix) have been used extensively in the clinical settings (e.g. Avolio *et al.* 2018; Safar *et al.* 2018). Increased wave reflection exerts its direct influence on arterial compliance through increased pressure amplitude (Li *et al.*, 2010). On the other hand, Aix has been shown to be not a direct correlate of arterial compliance (Kaya *et al.*, 2022). Methods of clinical measurements of vascular stiffness have been previously reviewed in several articles (e.g. Boutouyrie, 2008; Sakuragi and Abhayaratna, 2010).

The use of arterial elastance (E_{as}) is common in the analysis and interpretation of ventricular–arterial system interaction. It should be noted here that E_{as} differs from C, as E_{as} is a system property, whereas arterial compliance is a structural property (e.g. Li, 2000a, 2004; Kerkhof *et al.*, 2013).

Metrics based on a difference are not unique, as numerous combinations of primary data involved may yield the same value when subtracted, such as PP = $P_s - P_d$. Therefore, the introduction of a "companion" metric is mandatory for a comprehensive analysis (Kerkhof *et al.*, 2019a). This concept has been applied to arterial blood pressure data collected in children (Kerkhof *et al.*, 2019b) which documents the findings for PP and the associated PPC. PP has been incorporated in an expression for calculating total arterial compliance ($C_v = \text{SV}/\text{PP}$). Interestingly, P_d/P_s is inversely and nearly linearly associated with PP, as recently illustrated by Kerkhof *et al.* (2022).

References

Armentano, R, Simon, A, Levenson, J, Chau, NP, Megnien, JL and Pichel, R (1991) Mechanical pressure versus intrinsic effects of hypertension on large arteries in humans, *Hypertension* **18**, 657–664.

Atlas, GM and Li, JK-J (2009) Brachial artery differential characteristic impedance: Contributions from changes in Young modulus and diameter, *Cardiovasc. Eng.* **9**, 11–17.

Avolio, AP, Kuznetsova, T, Heyndrickx, GR, Kerkhof, PLM and Li, JK-J (2018) Arterial flow, pulse pressure and pulse wave velocity in men and women at various ages, in *Sex-Specific Analysis of Cardiovascular Function*, Advances in Experimental Biology and Medicine, Vol. 1065 (Springer, Cham), pp. 153–168.

Bahlmann, E, Cramariuc, D, Saeed, S, Chambers, JB, Nienaber, CA, Kuck, K-H, Lønnebakken, MT and Gerdts, E (2019) Low systemic arterial compliance is associated with increased cardiovascular morbidity and mortality in aortic valve stenosis, *Heart* **105**, 1507–1514.

Berger, DS and Li, JK-J (1990) Concurrent compliance reduction and increased peripheral resistance in the manifestation of isolated systolic hypertension, *Am. J. Cardiol.* **65**, 67–71.

Boutouyrie, P (2008) New techniques for assessing arterial stiffness, *Diabetes Metab.* **34**, S21–S26.

Chemla, D, Hébert, J-L, Coirault, C, Zamani, K, Suard, I, Colin, P and Lecarpentier, Y (1998) Total arterial compliance estimated by stroke volume-to-aortic pulse pressure ratio in humans, *Am. J. Physiol., Heart Circ. Physiol.* **274**, H500–H505.

Cox, RH (1975) Pressure dependence of the mechanical properties of arteries in vivo, *Am. J. Physiol.* **229**, 1371–1375.

Craim, D, Graf, SN, Armentano, RL and Barra, JG (2012) Vascular smooth muscle activation improves aortic compliance with respect to mechanical loading, *Cardiovasc. Eng. Technol.* **3**, 80–87.

de Simone, G, Roman, MJ, Koren, MJ, Mensah, GA, Ganau, A and Devereux, RB (1999) Stroke volume/pulse pressure ratio and cardiovascular risk in arterial hypertension, *Hypertension* **33**, 800–805.

Drzewiecki, G, Field, S, Mubarak, I and Li, JK-J (1997) Effect of vascular growth pattern on lumen area and compliance using a novel pressure-area model for collapsible vessels, *Am. J. Physiol., Heart Circ. Physiol.* **273**, H2030–H2043.

Fagard, RH, Pardaens, K, Staessen, JA and Thijs, L (2001) The pulse pressure-to-stroke index ratio predicts cardiovascular events and death in uncomplicated hypertension, *J. Am. Coll. Cardiol.* **38**, 227–231.

Fung, YC (1997) *Biomechanics: Circulation* (Springer-Verlag, New York).

Ghio, S, Morsolini, M, Corsico, A, Klersy, C, Mattiucci, G, Raineri, C, Scelsi, L, Vistarini, N, Visconti, LO and D'Armini, AM (2014) Pulmonary arterial compliance and exercise capacity after pulmonary endarterectomy, *Eur. Respir. J.* **43**, 1403–1409.

Goldwyn, RM and Watt, TB (1967) Arterial pressure pulse contour analysis via a mathematical model for the clinical quantification of human vascular properties, *IEEE Trans. Biomed. Eng.* **14**, 11–17.

Haluska, BA, Jeffries, L, Carlier, S and Marwick, TH (2010) Measurement of arterial distensibility and compliance to assess prognosis, *Atherosclerosis* **209**, 474–480.

Humphrey, JD (2013) *Cardiovascular Solid Mechanics: Cells, Tissues, and Organs* (Springer, New York).

Iantorno, S and Li, JK-J (1988) Compliance indices in the assessment of cardiac diseases, in *Proc Annu Int Conf IEEE Engineering in Medicine and Biology*, Vol. 10 (New Orleans, USA), pp. 247–248.

Ilercil, A, Zhu, Y, Wu, J, Li, JK-J, Lee, M and Nanna, M (1995) Computer model prediction of left ventricular hypertrophy based on the concept of a double loaded ventricle, *J. Am. Soc. Echocardiogr.* **8**, 383.

Kaya, M, Balasubramaniana, V, Patel, A, Ge, Y and Li, JK-J (2018) A novel compliance-pressure loop approach to quantify arterial compliance in systole and in diastole, *Comput. Biol. Med.* **99**, 98–106.

Kaya, M, Balasubramanian, V and Li, JK-J (2022) Inadequacy of augmentation index for monitoring arterial stiffness: Comparison with arterial compliance and other hemodynamic variables, *J. Cardiovasc. Eng. Technol.* **13**, 590–602.

Kerkhof, PLM, Li, JK-J and Heyndrickx, GR (2013) Effective arterial elastance and arterial compliance in heart failure patients with preserved ejection fraction, in *Proc 2013 35th Annu Int Conf IEEE Engineering in Medicine and Biology Society* (Osaka, Japan), pp. 691–694, doi:10.1109/EMBC.2013.6609594.

Kerkhof, PLM, Peace, RA and Handly, N (2019a) Ratiology and a complementary class of metrics for cardiovascular investigations, *Physiology (Bethesda)* **34**(4), 250–263, doi:10.1152/physiol.00056.2018.

Kerkhof, PLM, Konradi, AO, Shlyakhto, EV, Handly, N and Li, JK-J (2019b) Polar coordinate description of blood pressure measurements and implications for sex-specific and personalized analysis, in *Proc 2019 41st Annu Int Conf IEEE Engineering in Medicine and Biology Society* (Berlin, Germany), pp. 502–505, doi:10.1109/EMBC.2019.8857346.

Kerkhof, PLM, Diaz-Navarro, RA, Heyndrickx, GR, Konradi, AO, Shlyakhto, EV, Handly, N and Li, JK-J (2022) The ratio of diastolic and systolic arterial pressure is associated with pulse pressure, in *Proc 2022 44th Annu Int Conf IEEE Engineering in Medicine and Biology Society* (Glasgow, Scotland, UK), pp. 1–4, doi:10.1109/EMBC48229.2022.9871478.

Laskey, WK, Parker, HG, Ferrari, VA, Kussmal, WG and Noordergraaf, A (1990) Estimation of total systemic arterial compliance in humans, *J. Appl. Physiol.* **69**, 112–119.

Li, JK-J (1986) Comparative cardiac mechanics: Laplace's law, *J. Theor. Biol.* **118**, 339–343.

Li, JK-J (1987) *Arterial System Dynamics* (New York University Press, New York).

Li, JK-J (1996) *Comparative Cardiovascular Dynamics of Mammals* (CRC Press, New York).

Li, JK-J (1998) A new description of arterial function: The compliance-pressure loop, *Angiology, J. Vasc. Dis.* **49**, 543–548.

Li, JK-J (2000a) *The Arterial Circulation: Physical Principles and Clinical Applications* (Human Press (Springer), New York).

Li, JK-J (2000b) Scaling and invariants in cardiovascular biology, in J. H. Brown and G. B. West (eds.), *Scaling in Biology* (Oxford University Press, Oxford, UK), pp. 113–128.

Li, JK-J (2004) *Dynamics of the Vascular System* (World Scientific, Singapore).

Li, JK-J (2018a) *Dynamics of the Vascular System — Interaction with the Heart*, 2nd ed. (World Scientific, Singapore).

Li, JK-J (2018b) Arterial wall properties in men and women: Hemodynamic analysis and clinical implications, in *Sex-Specific Analysis of Cardiovascular Function*, Advances in Experimental Biology and Medicine, Vol. 1065 (Springer, Cham), pp. 291–306.

Li, JK-J, Melbin, J, Riffle, RA and Noordergraaf, A (1981) Pulse wave propagation, *Circ. Res.* **49**, 442–452.

Li, JK-J, Cui, T and Drzewiecki, G (1990) A nonlinear model of the arterial system incorporating a pressure-dependent compliance, *IEEE Trans. Biomed. Eng.* **BME-37**, 673–678.

Li, JK-J and Zhu, Y (1994) Arterial compliance and its pressure dependence in hypertension and vasodilation, *Angiology, J. Vasc. Dis.* **45**, 113–117.

Li, JK-J, Zhu, Y and Drzewiecki, G (1994) Pulse pressure is a significant determinant of arterial compliance in hypertension and vasodilation, *Circulation* **90**, 1166.

Li, JK-J, Zhu, JY and Nanna, M (1997) Computer modeling of the effects of aortic valve stenosis and arterial system afterload on left ventricular hypertrophy, *Comput. Biol. Med.* **27**, 477–485.

Li, JK-J, Zhu, Y, O'Hara, D and Khaw, K (2007) Allometric hemodynamic analysis of isolated systolic hypertension and aging, *Cardiovasc. Eng.* **7**, 135–139.

Li, JK-J, Zhu, Y and Geipel, PS (2010) Pulse pressure, arterial compliance and wave reflection under differential vasoactive and mechanical loading, *Cardiovasc. Eng.* **10**, 170–175.

Liu, Z, Brin, KP and Yin, FC (1986) Estimation of total arterial compliance: An improved method and evaluation of current methods, *Am. J. Physiol.* **251**, H588–H600.

Marcus, RH, Korcarz, C, McCray, G, Neumann, A, Murphy, M, Borow, K, Weinert, L, Bednarz, J, Gretler, DD and Spencer, KT (1994) Noninvasive method for determination of arterial compliance using Doppler echocardiography and subclavian pulse tracings validation and clinical application of a physiological model of the circulation, *Circulation* **89**, 2688–2699.

Matonick, J and Li, JK-J (2001) Pressure-dependent and frequency domain characteristics of the systemic arterial system, *Cardiovasc. Eng.* **1**, 21–29.

McVeigh, GE, Bratteli, CW, Morgan, DJ, Alinder, CM, Glasser, SP, Finkelstein, SM and Cohn, JN (1999) Age-related abnormalities in arterial compliance identified by pressure pulse contour analysis: Aging and arterial compliance, *Hypertension* **33**, 1392–1398.

Noordergraaf, A (1969) Hemodynamics, in H. P. Schwan (ed.), *Biological Engineering* (McGraw-Hill, New York), pp. 391–545.

Noordergraaf, A (2011) *Blood in Motion* (Springer, New York).

Papaioannou, TG, Protogerou, AD, Stergiopulos, N, Vardoulis, O, Stefanadis, C, Safar, M and Blacher, J (2014) Total arterial compliance estimated by a novel method and all-cause mortality in the elderly: The PROTEGER study, *Age (Dordr.)* **36**, 1555–1563.

Perret, F, Mooser, V, Hayoz, D, Tardy, Y, Meister, JJ, Etienne, JD, Farine, PA, Marazzi, A, Burnier, M and Nussberger, J (1991) Evaluation of arterial compliance-pressure curves: Effect of antihypertensive drugs, *Hypertension* **18**(4_Suppl II), 77–83.

Phan, TS, Li, JK-J, Segers, P, Koppula, MR, Akers, SR, Kuna, ST, Gislason, T, Pack, AI and Chirinos, JA (2016) Aging is associated with an earlier arrival of reflected waves without a distal shift in reflection sites, *J. Am. Heart Assoc.* **5**, e003733, doi:10.1161/JAHA.116.003733.

Resnick, LM, Militianu, D, Cunnings, AJ, Pipe, JG, Evelhoch, JL, Soulen, RL and Lester, MA (2000) Pulse waveform analysis of arterial compliance: Relation to other techniques, age, and metabolic variables, *Am. J. Hypertens.* **13**, 1243–1249.

Roman, MJ, Devereux, RB, Kizer, JR, Lee, ET, Galloway, JM, Ali, T, Umans, JG and Howard, BV (2007) Central pressure more strongly relates to vascular disease and outcome than does brachial pressure: The Strong Heart Study, *Hypertension* **50**, 197–203.

Safar, ME, Asmar, R, Benetos, A, Blacher, J, Boutouyrie, P, Lacolley, P, Laurent, S, Longon, G, Pannier, B, Protogerou, A, Regnault, V and French Study Group on Arterial Stiffness (2018) Interaction between hypertension and arterial stiffness: An expert reappraisal, *Hypertension* **72**, 796–805.

Sakuragi, S and Abhayaratna, WP (2010) Arterial stiffness: Methods of measurement, physiologic determinants and prediction of cardiovascular outcomes, *Int. J. Cardiol.* **138**, 112–118.

Stergiopulos, N, Segers, P and Westerhof, N (1999) Use of pulse pressure method for estimating total arterial compliance in vivo, *Am. J. Physiol.* **276**(2), H424–H428.

Somlyo, AP and Somlyo, AV (1968) Vascular smooth muscle, 1. Normal structure, pathology, biochemistry and biophysics, *Pharm. Rev.* **20**, 197–272.

Syeda, B, Gottsauner-Wolf, M, Denk, S, Pichler, P, Khorsand, A and Glogar, D (2003) Arterial compliance: A diagnostic marker for atherosclerotic plaque burden? *Am. J. Hypertens.* **16**, 356–362.

Thubrikar, MJ and Robicsek, S (1995) Pressure-induced arterial wall stress and atherosclerosis, *Ann. Thorac. Surg.* **59**, 1594–1603.

van Bortel, LM and Spek, JJ (1998) Influence of aging on arterial compliance, *J. Hum. Hypertens.* **12**, 583–586.

van Loo, C, Giudici, A and Spronck, B (2022) Potential adverse effects of vasodilatory antihypertensive medication on vascular stiffness in elderly individuals, *Hypertens. Res.* **45**, 2024–2027, doi:10.1038/s41440-022-01012-0.

Villard, C, Eriksson, P, Swedenborg, J and Hultgren, R (2014) Differences in elastin and elastolytic enzymes between men and women with abdominal aortic aneurysm, *Aorta* **2**, 179–185.

Wagenseil, JE and Mecham, RP (2012) Elastin in large artery stiffness and hypertension, *J. Cardiovasc. Transl. Res.* **5**, 264–273.

Watt, TB and Burrus, C (1976) Arterial pressure contour analysis for estimating human vascular properties, *J. Appl. Physiol.* **40**, 171–176.

Weizsacker, HW and Pascal, K (1982) Anisotropic passive properties of blood vessel walls, in Eds. T. Kenner, R. Busse and H. Hinghofer-Szalkay (eds.), *Cardiovascular System Dynamics: Models and Measurements* (Plenum Press, New York), pp. 347–362.

Wells, SM, Langeille, BL and Adamson, SL (1998) In vivo and in vitro mechanical properties of the sheep in thoracic aorta in the perinatal period and adulthood, *Am. J. Physiol.* **274**, H1749–H1760.

Westerhof, N and Noordergraaf, A (1970) Arterial viscoelasticity: A generalized model, *J. Biomech.* **3**, 357–379.

CHAPTER 2

Noninvasive Brachial Artery Mechanics and Endothelial Function[a]

Gary Drzewiecki

Department of Biomedical Engineering,
School of Engineering Rutgers,
The State University of New Jersey, 599 Taylor Road,
Piscataway, NJ 08854, USA
garydrz@soe.rutgers.edu

It has been recognized that endothelial dysfunction is an early indication of Arterial disease. Endothelial function can be noninvasively evaluated by Inducing a temporary increase in blood flow and then observing the degree of vasodilation response or flow-mediated dilation. Impaired flow mediated vasodilation is then an indication of impaired endothelium. Vascular ultrasound Imaging has been the typical approach to access vasodilation by flow-mediated dilation most often at the brachial artery. Together with other measures of cardiovascular risk, the flow-mediated dilation response provides a very early noninvasive screen for cardiovascular disease. The skill and equipment required for brachial artery ultrasound imaging have limited the use of flow-mediated dilation as a routine medical test. Moreover, it has been recognized that other vascular parameters such as vessel size and blood pressure may influence the test itself.

We have introduced a potential solution to the routine measurement of flow-mediated dilation by Analyzing the response of a simple occlusive arm cuff to obtain the Brachial Artery diameter in a noninvasive way. The analysis for occlusive cuff Plethysmography was provided here in a calibrated manner. This approach is an alternative to ultrasound flow-mediated dilation testing. It requires no special operator skills and may be automated for precision.

Two experimental evaluations of the proposed cuff method are provided. First, The cuff-based brachial diameters were compared to Ultrasound obtained diameters. Second, as a sensitivity test, the cuff-based dilation test was used to measure the dilation response of several subjects to blood sugar loading. For further evaluation, the cuff-based measurements were applied to a mechanical model of the brachial artery to reveal a standard error of estimate less than 5%. The results show that the cuff-based diameters compare well to those obtained via ultrasound imaging. Moreover, the cuff-based dilation testing showed

---

[a]This article was previously published in *World Scientific Annual Review of Biomechanics*. Vol: 1, (2023) 2330002 (14 pages).

the expected reduction in endothelial function response due to a blood sugar load. Additionally, cuff-based flow-mediated dilation testing provides measurements as a function of the subject blood pressure, which Ultrasound generally cannot.

Keywords: Noninvasive endothelial function; flow-mediated dilation; cardiovascular risk; occlusive cuff plethysmography.

1. Biomechanics of the Human Brachial Artery

1.1. *Arterial pressure–area relationship*

The brachial artery (BA) is a flexible structure that exhibits wall stretch while pressurized. The degree of stretch then determines the vessel diameter, assuming a circular shape. Stretch is further determined by the vascular wall properties such as thickness, elasticity, and smooth muscle tone. When the vessel has external pressure applied, such as with the application of a pressure cuff, the artery may be forced to partly collapse. This entire range of vessel function can be depicted by plotting the vessel lumen area versus its transmural pressure, where transmural pressure is the internal pressure minus the external pressure. Figure 1 provides an example of a typical brachial artery pressure–area relationship.

The brachial artery lumen area–pressure for a single subject is shown in Figure 1. Data points were obtained noninvasively via cuff plethysmography (CP). The solid line is a mechanical model [Eq. (1)] fit to the data. The regions of stretch and collapse are modeled below in Eq. (1), where the left term represents arterial distension and stretch, while the right term is vessel collapse during negative

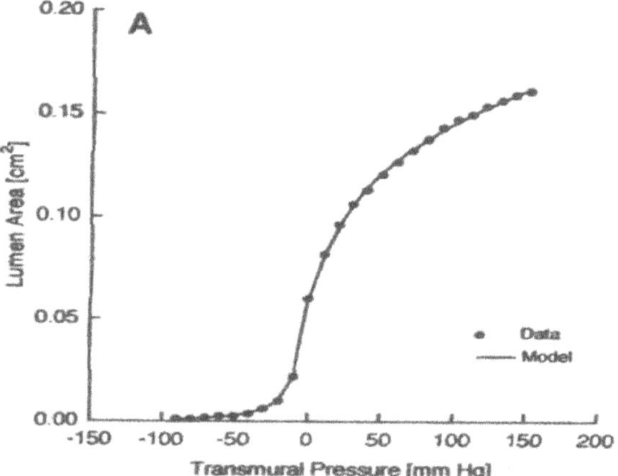

Fig. 1.   Brachial artery pressure–area relationship.

Source: Reproduced from Drzewiecki and Pilla (1998).

transmural pressure. The lumen area is A, and transmural pressure is P_t. P_b is an empirical parameter that represents the pressure at which the vessel buckles. The parameter A_b is the lumen area at which vessel buckling occurs. All parameters are obtained via a nonlinear fit to vessel pressure–area data. Thus, Figure 1 and Eq. (1) provide an overall summary of vessel mechanics in one function,

$$Pt = a\left(e^{\frac{b(A-A_b)}{A_b}} - 1\right) - E\left(\left(\frac{A_b}{A}\right)^n - 1\right) + P_b.$$ (1)

1.2. *Smooth muscle effect*

The data of Figure 1 were for the condition of a vessel at rest. That is, the vascular smooth muscle was at its resting level of muscle tone. The pressure–area curve also provides a convenient display of smooth muscle effect on an artery. The human brachial artery was permitted to dilate from its normal rest condition as shown in Figure 2.

The brachial artery lumen area versus transmural pressure was obtained on a single normal subject. Transmural pressure is the mean arterial pressure-cuff pressure. Dots are actual data samples for the transmural pressure. Pre-dilation

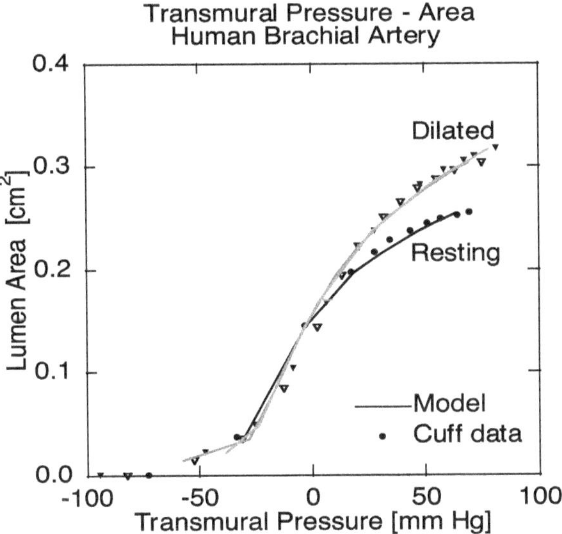

Fig. 2.   The brachial artery lumen area versus transmural pressure is obtained on a single normal subject. Transmural pressure is mean arterial pressure-cuff pressure. Dots are actual data samples for the transmural pressure. Pre-dilation is the rest curve. Post-dilation is the dilated curve. The solid line curve is a nonlinear model fit to the data points. Data points are obtained using the noninvasive cuff plethysmography method.

is the control curve. Post-dilation is the dilated curve. The solid line curve is a nonlinear model fit to the data using Eq. (1). Note that the biomechanic arterial model applies equally well to the rest and vasodilated conditions. Likewise, the pressure–lumen area plot is a complete way of analyzing the vessel mechanics in a single graph such as in this case where the smooth muscle effect is of interest. Hence, in a single graph the mechanical geometry and function may be observed as well as the biological function. This approach will be applied later in this paper to study the endothelial function.

Data points were obtained using the cuff plethysmography method.

1.3. *Measurement of brachial pressure–area relationship*

Understanding that the pressure–area relationship offers a general biomechanical description of vessel function, it is desirable to measure this aspect of vessel function. An *in-vitro* experimental method was originally introduced by Drzewiecki *et al.* (1997). But to be clinically practical, a noninvasive approach to measure the pressure–area data is sought. Occlusive arm cuff plethysmography serves that purpose well and is described next.

1.4. *Occlusive cuff plethysmography for noninvasive arterial mechanics*

Arterial plethysmography has been employed to obtain the arterial pulse waveform (Nabeel *et al.*, 2017). However, by definition, a plethysmograph sensor measures the arterial volume and thereby the pulse pressure indirectly. Hence a calibrated plethysmograph provides arterial pulse volume. For example, there is the optical pulse plethysmograph (Seo *et al.*, 2016), which is also an output of the pulse oximeter. Since plethysmography provides arterial volume change in a noninvasive way, some researchers have employed it as a nonultrasound approach to obtain vessel lumen area. For example, Drzewiecki *et al.* (1993) modeled an occlusive arm cuff's mechanics to investigate its use as a volume sensor. This work revealed the functional relationship between cuff pressure and volume. Moreover, an occlusive cuff has the additional advantage of permitting the arterial transmural pressure to be altered experimentally. A typical recording of the cuff pressure pulse versus cuff pressure is provided in Figure 3.

Although Figure 3 illustrates cuff pressure and cuff pressure oscillations, the oscillations in cuff pressure, dP, are converted to volume using cuff compliance knowledge. So, the arterial volume pulse dV is then determined as

$$dV = C_{\text{cuff}} \times dP. \tag{2}$$

Since the occlusive cuff responds to arterial volume pulsations, the cuff pressure pulse may be converted to a volume pulse using Eq. (2) and knowledge of the

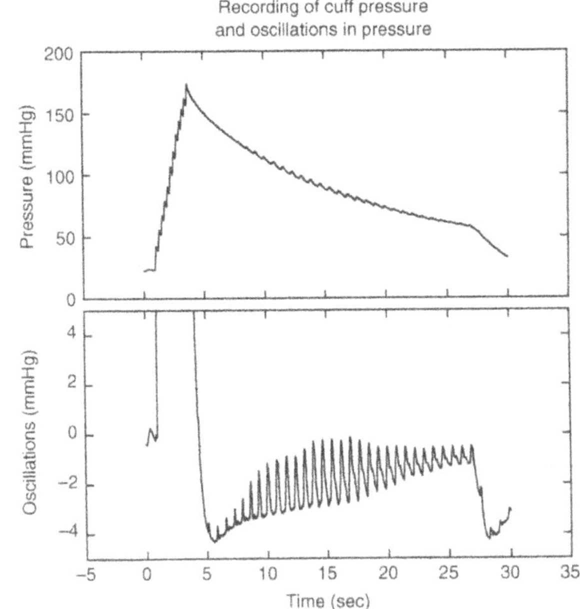

Fig. 3. Top panel: Occlusive cuff pressure recording while on a subject's upper arm during an inflation–deflation cycle. Bottom panel: The brachial artery pulse derived from the high-pass-filtered cuff pressure of the top panel. The filtered oscillations are equivalent to the arterial volume pulse reproduced from (Drzewiecki *et al.*, 1993).

cuff compliance C_{cuff}. Next, we convert the raw cuff data into the arterial transmural pressure–lumen area curve as in Figure 2. Then, on a beat-by-beat basis, the cuff data is recorded as pulse volume $[dV_i, TP]$, where i denotes the pulse beat number and dV is obtained from the cuff pressure pulse dP and C_{cuff} using Eq. (2). Every pulse pair is then analyzed to obtain the brachial artery lumen area TP curve as in Figure 2. This final arterial volume result is obtained by mathematical integration of the volume pulses dV with respect to TP as follows:

$$V = \int dV dTP. \tag{3}$$

Since the data points are obtained as a list of $[dV, TP]$ pairs, the integration is numerically computed via a numerical integration algorithm. The initial condition of this integration is treated as arterial volume is zero so that $V = 0$. By starting the integration at high cuff pressure and referring to Figure 3, high cuff pressure occurs at about the time of 5 s. It can be seen that the cuff pulses are relatively small at this time. This means that the arterial volume is nearly zero in this range since the artery is nearly completely collapsed. This analysis procedure allows a complete synthesis of the arterial pressure–lumen area curve. Hence, noninvasive cuff pressure data may be converted into the arterial pressure–lumen area curve to provide an overview of the vessel biomechanics. This method will be applied later in this paper to noninvasively study vascular biology.

2. Vascular Biology

As portrayed so far, the artery is not a passive elastic tube. Instead, the arterial wall is a composite of passive structure fibers, smooth muscle, and endothelial tissue. The activation of vascular smooth muscle serves to regulate local blood flow by means of altering the vessel diameter. The endothelial tissue lines the inner wall of the blood vessels and is therefore in contact with the blood. It serves to protect the vascular wall and also communicate and modulate smooth muscle tone.

3. Endothelial Function

As shown in Figure 4, the endothelium is in contact with blood flow and serves as a barrier to blood and the arterial wall smooth muscle. The blood flow shear of the endothelium stimulates normal endothelium to release nitrous oxide, NO, to the arterial wall. NO causes the smooth muscle to relax and the vessel to vasodilate.

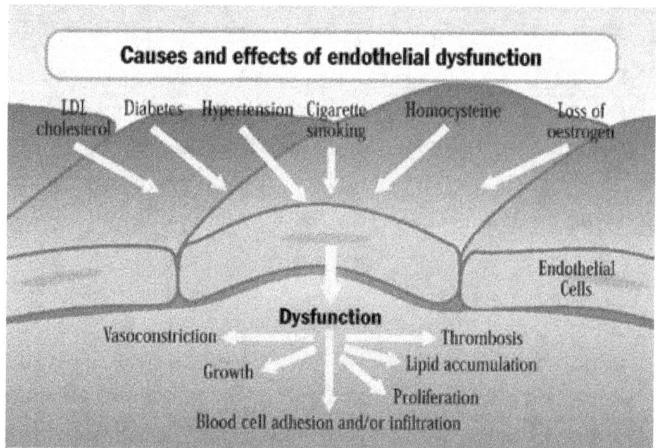

Fig. 4.   Illustration of a layer of endothelial cells that line the inner wall of an artery. The blood flow side is above the cells where various sources of cell injury may occur. The layer below the cells is the arterial wall consisting of structural tissue and smooth muscle.

3.1. *Cardiovascular disease and endothelial function*

In the presence of cardiovascular disease, the endothelial function is impaired. The dysfunctional responses are also shown in Figure 4. The net result is that smooth muscle relaxation is reduced. This is primarily due to the reduced NO that is released by the endothelium (Deanfield *et al.*, 2007).

3.2. *Endothelial dysfunction and artery disease*

The presence of cardiovascular disease may be detected indirectly by measuring the smooth muscle relaxation response to blood flow which indirectly tests the endothelial function. The measurable response is that arterial vasodilation due to blood flow increase is reduced in the presence of cardiovascular disease (Thijssen *et al.*, 2019). This is defined as the flow-mediated dilation (FMD) response (Celermajer *et al.*, 1992).

It is therefore desirable to measure the FMD response of an artery to indirectly detect the presence of endothelial damage due to vascular disease. To do this noninvasively in humans, first a blood flow increase is required. Second, a means of measuring the arterial diameter in the baseline state and following the flow increase is required. Various methods have been developed to noninvasively measure FMD in the brachial artery. They are now reviewed here.

4. Noninvasive Measurement of Endothelial Function by FMD

4.1. *Brachial Artery Ultrasound Imaging*

The method of ultrasound brachial artery FMD was developed to examine the brachial artery noninvasively (Vogel, 2001). The brachial artery was chosen due to its relative proximity to the heart. Moreover, brachial artery disease correlates well with coronary artery disease (CAD) (Deanfield *et al.*, 2007). Therefore, impaired brachial endothelial function should be a good risk factor for coronary artery disease (The CARDIoGRAMplusC4D Consortium *et al.*, 2013). The method of ultrasound FMD procedure is as follows. First, the arterial resting diameter D_{rest} is imaged using ultrasound imaging. Second, a blood flow increase is accomplished by occluding blood flow for a brief period, about 5 min, to cause an increase in arm blood flow via the reactive hyperemia response. Then, vessel diameter is imaged again following occlusion to observe vessel vasodilation diameter D_{vaso}. The %FMD is then defined according to Eq. (4) as the percent change in diameter,

$$(D_{vaso} - D_{rest})/D_{rest} \times 100\% = \%FMD. \tag{4}$$

4.2. *Cuff plethysmography-BA testing*

CP may be used instead of Brachial Artery Ultrasound Imaging (BAUI) to obtain the brachial artery diameters as described in Figs. 2 and 3. Experiments were performed to obtain the BA diameters of eight normal subjects (Whitt and Drzewiecki, 2010). The same subjects were recorded using the arm cuff plethysmography method and the data were analyzed as described in the methods to obtain cuff BA diameters for direct comparison. Comparative testing was performed using Doppler ultrasonography as the control measurement. The eight subjects for the experiments included five healthy women and three healthy men ranging from 23 years to 57 years of age. Independent sociometric blood subjects in pressure measurements were performed on all subjects using both an automated oscillometer and the cuff plethysmograph. Two trials were performed: one for the BA resting condition and a second trial following FMD. A scatter plot provides BA diameter by ultrasound versus BA diameter by CP. Cuff plethysmography shows the final experimental results and a linear fit to each dataset for all can be observed in Figure 5.

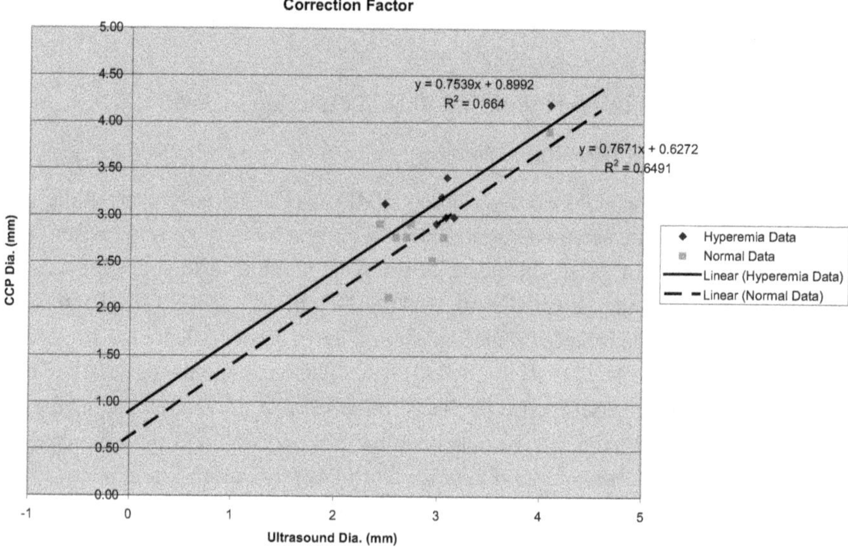

Fig. 5.   BA diameter obtained by plethysmography versus ultrasound imaging for each subject.
Source: Reproduced from. Whitt and Drzewiecki (2010).

The straight lines in Figure 5 are linear fits to each data. The linear regression equations are shown next to each linear fit. The data reveal that cuff plethysmography measures of arterial diameter can be a viable alternative to BAUI-based %FMD tested.

4.3. *Indirect approaches to FMD testing*

4.3.1. *Digital volume pulse method*

Other indirect measures of FMD have been proposed that employ more peripheral measures of arterial response to blood flow at the digital artery, e.g., by measuring the finger pulse or finger temperature.

Such an alternative noninvasive approach to measuring FMD was developed by (Bonetti *et al.*, 2004). They chose to measure %FMD at the fingertip instead of at the brachial artery. To do this, a volume sensor is placed at a fingertip to record pulsations at a digit. As in other approaches, a temporary cuff tourniquet is applied to the brachial artery for 5 min to prevent brachial blood flow. The peripheral volume pulse at the finger is then recorded before and after flow occlusion. A sample finger pulse recording is shown in Figure 6.

The key observation in Figure 6 is that the post-occlusion volume pulse is reduced as compared with the pre-occlusion pulse. Although this measurement

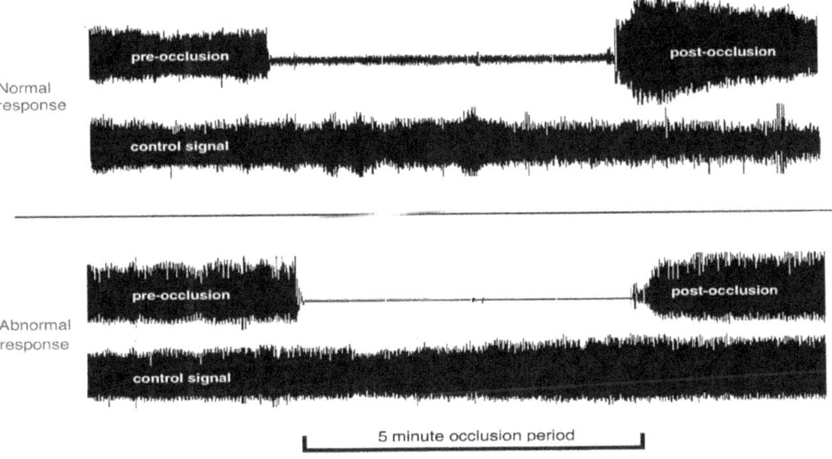

Fig. 6.   Sample finger pulse recordings before, during, and after brachial artery occlusion. Two patients are shown: one normal and a second with known coronary artery disease.

Source: Reproduced from (Bonetti *et al.*, 2004).

is performed at a peripheral vessel, the researchers suggest that the response is equivalent to a brachial artery FMD response. This device has been evaluated on a large subject population and is currently FDA-approved. The instrument is offered by the Itamar Corporation for clinical use.

4.4. *Finger thermal response method for FMD*

In a similar manner to the finger pulse method of FMD, the fingertip temperature was proposed to be used as an indirect measure of peripheral blood flow prior to and after a flow occlusion (Naghavi *et al.*, 2022). Sample finger temperature response curves are shown in Figure 7.

Sample finger temperature responses before and after blood flow occlusion are shown in Figure 7. A rebound in finger temperature to at least pre-occlusion levels is considered a healthy endothelial function. This method has shown good correlation with CAD in a study of over 100 subjects. The instrument is now commercially available from the Endothelix Corp. While this measurement correlates well with CAD, it does not directly measure %FMD as originally described by a change in brachial artery diameter. Instead, they are recording the flow changes due to brachial artery dilation. Nevertheless, these instruments are noninvasive and require minimal skill to operate. In spite of their simplicity, BAUI remains to be the standard for FMD large-scale experimental studies (The CARDIoGRAMplusC4D Consortium *et al.*, 2013).

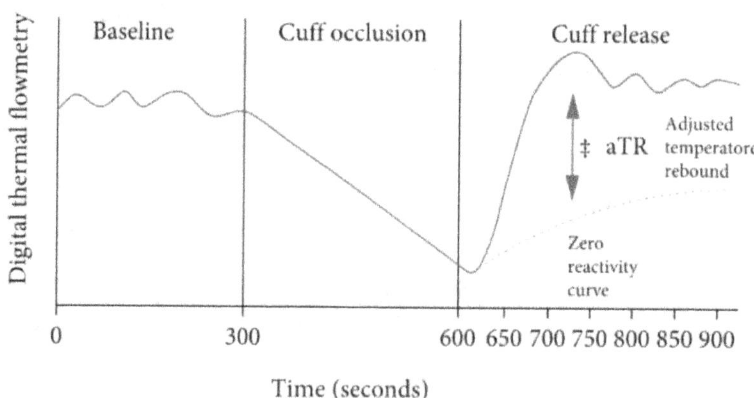

Fig. 7.   FMD via finger thermal responses. The finger temperatures are shown before, during, and after occlusion. The dotted curve indicates a poor response and the possible detection of coronary artery disease.

Source: Reproduced from (Naghavi *et al.*, 2022).

5. Independent Sensitivity to Endothelial Function and FMD

5.1. *True endothelial function, CAD, and FMD variability*

Any of the methods described so far depend on their reliability in accurately responding to FMD alone with the exclusion of other factors. Some studies have revealed that FMD via BAUI is influenced by brachial artery diameter and blood pressure. This makes it difficult to identify a specific value of FMD that can be used for diagnostic purposes. As a result of this issue, FMD must be specified as a range of values considered to be healthy and those that are statistically correlated with CAD. Some common values of FMD for various subject groups are shown in Figure 8. Ultrasound %FMD procedure has been refined and standardized (Corretti *et al.*, 2002). A sample of %FMD ultrasound data is shown in Figure 8. It is clear that increased cardiovascular risk also results in a lower average %FMD in all groups studied. It is this good correlation of %FMD that makes this test of endothelial function interesting.

In each case in Figure 8, the pre-dilation control is shown. For the children group, FH indicates hypercholesterolemia. For adult subjects, %FMD in smoking groups and known CAD are shown. The horizontal bar denotes the mean value for the group. While it is clear that FMD offers a range of values, on average, a %FMD of less than 7% provides significant indication of the presence of CAD.

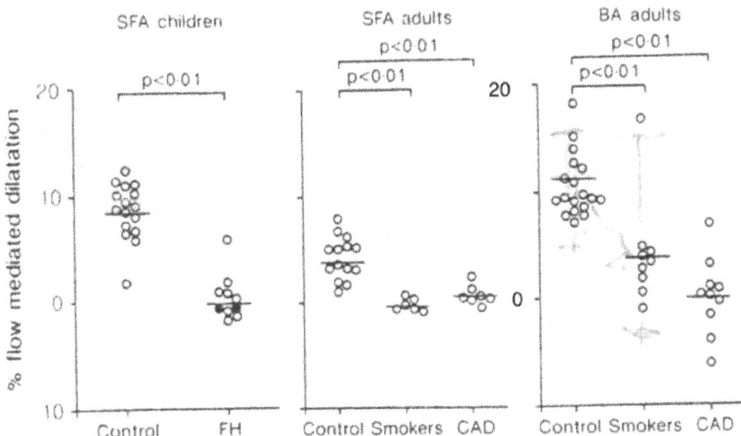

Fig. 8.   Ultrasound %FMD data obtained in 16 subjects: for children femoral artery (left panel), adult femoral artery (middle panel), and adult brachial artery (right panel). Here, FH denotes hypercholesterolemia.

Source: Reproduced from (Celermajer *et al.*, 1992).

While the %FMD experiments by BAUI can be applied to group studies where the subject numbers are sufficiently large to attain significant results, it is desirable to reduce %FMD variability so that it may be applied to small groups and individuals. Of first consideration is the variability due to the ultrasound imaging and operator accuracy. In (Celermajer *et al.*, 1992) study discussed above, using a 7-MHz imaging system, it was found that the instrumental error was only 1.7%. This is significantly less than the average %FMD of 7–10%. This next leads to other factors that need to be considered as sources of variability and other factors that may be confounding the measurement of % FMD.

5.2. *Diameter effect (vessel size)*

We consider next the effect of brachial artery size on FMD. In an artery, muscle length is proportionate to vessel diameter assuming a circular vessel. So, to normalize the effect of muscle length, the smooth muscle contractility is approximated as the percentage change in diameter. Unfortunately, normalizing the vessel dilation is not completely successful due to the nonlinearity of the muscle force–length curve. This is illustrated in Figure 9 where %FMD is shown versus the vessel initial diameter; this figure demonstrates that %FMD is inversely related to vessel diameter, showing that the usual FMD normalization is not capable of completely eliminating vessel diameter as a factor that alters %FMD.

5.3. *Blood pressure effect on FMD*

All tests of %FMD that have been reviewed here do not correct for the subject's blood pressure.

For example, referring to the BAUI method, BAUI is typically performed at the subject's resting blood pressure. Therefore, any influence of blood pressure on the FMD test is not corrected for (Park *et al.*, 2019) have shown that hypertension is correlated with reduced %FMD using BAUI. Similarly, the peripheral pulse methods of FMD suffer from this same problem. Alternatively, the FMD method of cuff plethysmography permits correction of blood pressure on FMD. This is possible since cuff plethysmography determines FMD versus transmural arterial pressure as opposed to absolute pressure. Hence, any subject may be measured at the same transmural pressure.

To illustrate, a cuff plethysmography study is provided next. Moreover, a complete range of pressure–area data allows for model-based analysis to be implemented. Model-based analysis affords an additional reduction in the variability of the data.

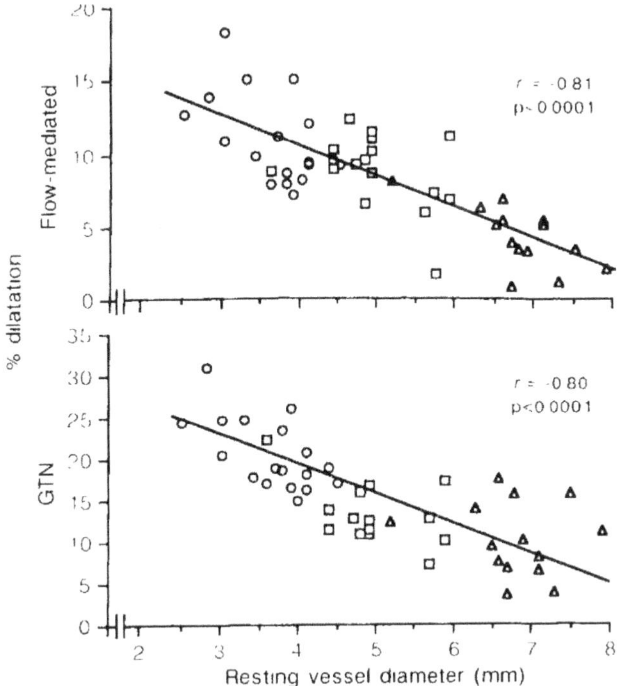

Fig. 9.   Ultrasound %FMD is shown versus the brachial artery pre-dilation diameter. %FMD is inversely related to vessel diameter. The solid line is the linear fit to the data points.

Source: Reproduced from (Celermajer *et al.*, 1992).

5.4. *Model-based analysis of FMD*

Six subjects were recorded using cuff plethysmography to obtain pressure–area data for the resting and FMD conditions. These data were input to the biomechanical BA model of Eq. (1). The model parameters were all obtained using MATLAB nonlinear regression. The nonlinear fit was performed for rest and dilated conditions to determine if the model could represent both states. The subjects were all free of cardiovascular disease and aged from 20 years to 50 years. A single-subject dataset is provided in Figure 10. IRB approval was obtained for this study performed at Rutgers University (IRB Pro20170002078). The full data is reported by Distefano (2018). The solid curve is a nonlinear fit to the vessel mechanical model of Eq. (1). Standard error of estimate was less than 5% for all subjects for both the rest and dilated conditions. Since this method allows data to be plotted as a function of pressure, it is clear that FMD is dependent on blood pressure. Model-based analysis results in considerably less variability of the data.

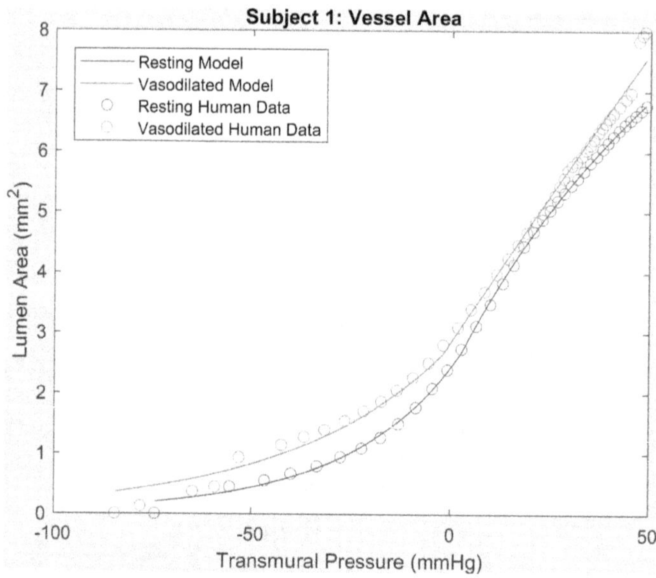

Fig. 10.   Single representative subject's pressure–lumen area data. Circle points are for the cuff plethysmograph data and the solid lines are the model fit to each dataset. The upper curve is the FMD condition. The lower curve is the resting BA condition. Blood pressure dependence of the data is evident for both curves.

Source: Reproduced from (Distefano, 2018).

5.5. *Sugar sensitivity*

It was lastly desirable to determine if the cuff plethysmography is sensitive to actual changes in BA endothelial function. A noninvasive experiment was used to alter endothelial function utilizing sugar loading several subjects and observing their FMD response using the cuff plethysmography method. Seven undergraduate student subjects were measured using the cuff plethysmograph first to obtain their control values of %FMD. The subject then consumed 100 g of sugar in the form of 0.94 L of a Snapple sugary beverage, giving them a limit of half an hour to consume the drinks and half an hour after they finish the drinks to absorb the sugar into the bloodstream. The FMD via cuff plethysmography was then repeated. The % changes in FMD with sugar loads are shown in Figure 11 for all subjects. There was a typical decrease in FMD for most subjects. ANOVA of this data confirmed a significant reduction in FMD to $p < 0.05$ versus the control FMD with an average of $-8.5+/-5.7\%$ reduction in FMD. Hence, the level of blood sugar during an FMD test may significantly affect an individual subject's %FMD value. This experiment confirms the sensitivity of the measured response to vascular function.

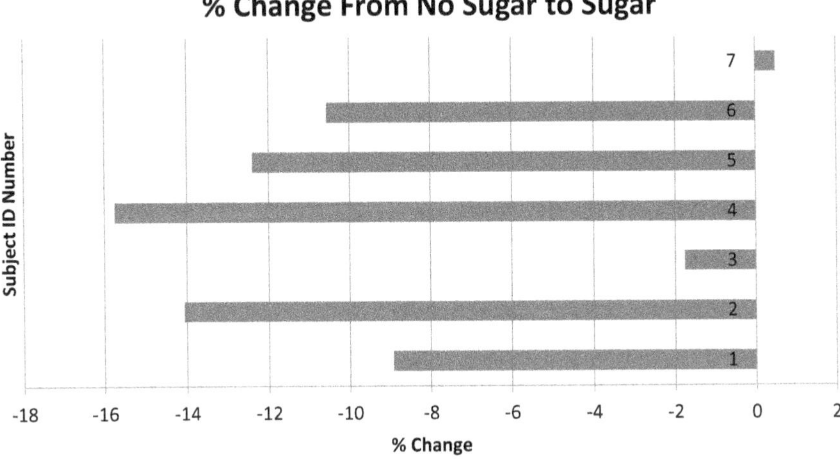

Fig. 11. Experimental changes in FMD in response to sugar loading for seven subjects. %FMD measurements are obtained using noninvasive cuff plethysmography.

Mah *et al.* (2011) have found a simlar impairment of endothelial function by blood sugar.

6. Summary

The flow mediation response was introduced as a means of noninvasively detecting the dysfunction of arterial endothelial function. Moreover, impaired endothelial function is associated with the presence of vascular disease. The brachial artery is an import site for the noninvasive testing of flow-mediated dilation. Furthermore, brachial artery disease is well correlated with coronary artery disease. Initially, ultrasound imaging has been the standard approach to measure %FMD. Other recent methods test FMD at the digital artery by means of pulse plethysmography and finger temperature. Some digital plethysmography device has become FDA-approved. Due to large variability of the test, FMD testing via ultrasound imaging has remained the standard for FMD studies. It was shown here that several factors that affect FMD may contribute to the variability of the test such as vessel size, blood pressure, and blood sugar level. The cuff plethysmography method of FMD was also reviewed and has the advantage of blood pressure correction. Finally, striving to ensure that the FMD test is a true independent test will increase its adoption as a routine clinical measurement. Model-based methods may help in this area.

References

Bonetti, PO, Pumper, GM, Higano, ST, Holmes, DR, Kuvin, JT and Lerman, A (2004) Noninvasive identification of patients with early coronary atherosclerosis by assessment of digital reactive hyperemia, *J. Am. Coll. Cardiol.* **44**(11), 2137–2141, doi:10.1016/j.jacc.2004.08.062.

Celermajer, DS, Sorensen, KE, Gooch, VM, Spiegelhalter, DJ, Miller, OI, Sullivan, ID, Lloyd, JK and Deanfield, JE (1992) Non-invasive detection of endothelial dysfunction in children and adults at risk of atherosclerosis, *Lancet* **340**(8828), 1111–1115, doi:10.1016/0140-6736(92)93147-f.

Corretti, MC, Anderson, TJ, Benjamin, EJ, Celermajer, D, Charbonneau, F, Creager, MA, Deanfield, J, Drexler, H, Garhard-Herman, M, Herrington, D, Vallance, P, Vita, J, Vogel, R and International Brachial Artery Reactivity Task Force (2002) Guidelines for the ultrasound assessment of endothelial-dependent flow-mediated vasodilation of the brachial artery: A report of the International Brachial Artery Reactivity Task Force, *J. Am. Coll. Cardiol.* **39**(2), 257–265, doi:10.1016/s0735-1097(01)01746-6.

Deanfield, JE, Halcox, JP and Rabelink, TJ (2007) Endothelial function and dysfunction: Testing and clinical relevance, *Circulation* **115**(10), 1285–1295, doi:10.1161/ CIRCU-LATIONAHA.106.652859.

Drzewiecki, G, Bansal, V, Karam, E, Hood, R and Apple, H (1993) Mechanics of the occlusive arm cuff and its application as a volume sensor, *IEEE Trans. Biomed. Eng.* **40**(7), 704–708, doi:10.1109/10.237700.

Drzewiecki, G, Field, S, Moubarak, I and Li, JK (1997) Vessel growth and collapsible pressure-area relationship, *Am. J. Physiol.* **273**(4), H2030–H2043, doi:10.1152/ajpheart.1997.273.4.H2030.

Drzewiecki, G and Pilla, JJ (1998) Noninvasive measurement of the human brachial artery pressure-area relation in collapse and hypertension, *Ann. Biomed. Eng.* **26**(6), 965–974, URL https://www.ncbi.nlm.nih.gov/pubmed/9846935.

Mah, E, Noh, SK, Ballard, KD, Matos, ME, Volek, JS and Bruno, RS (2011) Postprandial hyperglycemia impairs vascular endothelial function in healthy men by inducing lipid peroxidation and increasing asymmetric dimethylarginine:arginine, *J. Nutr.* **141**(11), 1961–1968, doi:10.3945/jn.111.144592.

Nabeel, PM, Joseph, J and Sivaprakasam, M (2017) A magnetic plethysmograph probe for local pulse wave velocity measurement, *IEEE Trans. Biomed. Circuits Syst.* **11**(5), 1065–1076, doi:10.1109/TBCAS.2017.2733622.

Park, K-H, Park, WJ, Han, SJ, Kim, H-S, Jo, SH, Kim, S-A and Suh, SW (2019) Association between intra-arterial invasive central and peripheral blood pressure and endothelial function (assessed by flow-mediated dilatation) in stable coronary artery disease, *Am. J. Hypertens.* **32**(10), 953–959.

Seo, E, Sazi, T, Togawa, M, Nagata, O, Murakami, M, Kojima, S and Seo, Y (2016) A portable infrared photoplethysmograph: heartbeat of *Mytilus galloprovincialis* analyzed by MRI and application to *Bathymodiolus septemdierum*, *Biol Open* **5**(11), 1752–1757, doi:10.1242/bio.020909.

The CARDIoGRAMplusC4D Consortium *et al.* (2013) Large-scale association analysis identifies new risk loci for coronary artery disease, *Nat. Genet.* **45**(1), 25–33, doi:10.1038/ng.2480.

Thijssen, DHJ, Bruno, RM, van Mil, A, Holder, SM, Faita, F, Greyling, A, Zock, PL, Taddei, S, Deanfield, JE, Luscher, T, Green, DJ and Ghiadoni, L (2019) Expert consensus and evidence-based recommendations for the assessment of flow-mediated dilation in humans, *Eur. Heart J.* **40**(30), 2534–2547, doi:10.1093/eurheartj/ehz350.

Vogel, RA (2001) Measurement of endothelial function by brachial artery flow-mediated vasodilation, *Am. J. Cardiol.* **88**(2A), 31E–34E, doi:10.1016/s0002-9149(01)01764-7.

Whitt, MD and Drzewiecki, GM (2010) Vascular mechanics in artificial and human arteries, in *Biomedical Engineering Principles of the Bionic Man*, Series on Bioengineering and Biomedical Engineering, Vol. 5 (World Scientific, Singapore), pp. 235–280.

CHAPTER 3

Analysis and Interpretation of Primary and Derived Data Sets in Cardiology[a]

Peter L. M. Kerkhof[*,††], John K.-J. Li[†], Rienzi A. Diaz-Navarro[‡,§], Guy R. Heyndrickx[¶],
Theo J. C. Faes[*], Francesco Tona[‖] and Neal Handly[**]

Department of Radiology and Nuclear Medicine,
Amsterdam University Medical Centers Location VUmc, Amsterdam, The Netherlands

†*Department of Biomedical Engineering, Rutgers University, Piscataway, NJ, USA*

‡*Department of Medicine, Universidad de Valparaíso, Valparaíso, Chile*

§*Cardiovascular Physiology Laboratory,*
Universidad de Valparaíso, Valparaíso, Chile

¶*Cardiovascular Center, OLV Clinic, Aalst, Belgium*

‖*Department of Cardiac, Thoracic and Vascular Sciences,*
University of Padova, Padova, Italy

**Department of Emergency Medicine,*
Drexel University College of Medicine, Philadelphia, PA, USA
††*plm.kerkhof@amsterdamumc.nl*

Investigators collect data and present them in a way that offers the best insight regarding the questions at hand. To facilitate understanding of certain aspects, it may occasionally be useful to rearrange primary data and formulate them as derived variables. For example, the travel distance divided by the invested time yields average velocity (as m/s). Problems may arise when interpreting ratios that fail to have a physical dimension. For example, current TV-sets have a fixed ratio for height and width, implying that we need an additional detail to define its size. Size then is determined by the diagonal, which can be calculated from the two sides using the Pythagorean theorem. Similarly, paired hemodynamic variables may be expressed as ratios. Again, a fixed ratio may refer to a variety of underlying primary data which require consideration if the ratio is unitless. In this survey, we evaluate several derived metrics commonly used in cardiovascular studies, and offer comprehensive analysis strategies.

Keywords: End-systolic volume; ejection fraction; blood pressure; fractional flow reserve; coronary flow reserve; augmentation index; ratiology; left ventricle.

---

††Corresponding author.
[a]This article was previously published in *World Scientific Annual Review of Biomechanics*. Vol: 1, (2023) 2330003 (23 pages).

1. Introduction to the Nature of Derived Metrics

Various clinically relevant quantities are measured as a data pair, and this combination typically refers to maximum and minimum values. Such a two-level approach particularly applies to cardiology and hemodynamics where many phenomena result from the phasic nature of the pumping heart. For example, systolic blood pressure (SBP) and diastolic blood pressure (DBP) are recorded in unison and concern a primary (or direct) data set. Baseline measurements may be compared to those obtained after medical intervention or during longitudinal studies, and can be analyzed, e.g. to predict the impact of risk factors on specific outcome measures.

Interestingly, in many biomedical disciplines/areas a tendency can be discerned where, mostly for convenience, investigators try to capture the bulk of multi-level information within a single composite metric (Kerkhof and Fu, 2022). The new index is often obtained by creating a mathematical construct built on an attractive arrangement/manipulation of the original data with preference for high-profile candidate variables that are characteristic of the focus of the study (Kerkhof *et al.*, 2019c). Thus, primary (direct) data are converted into derived data aiming to "reduce complexity" and thus promoting practical insight. The desired strategy perhaps resembles the familiar ease of interpreting a single variable such as body temperature, which features a well-defined normal range, a subfebrile state, and a frankly elevated high-grade fever, sometimes at life-threatening levels.

Several of those ambitious "reduction" efforts have resulted in the study of the mere difference, yielding pulse pressure (PP) which equals (SBP–DBP) in the study of arterial blood pressure-related risk factors. Also, the mean value of arterial pressure (MAP) or even the ratio (SBP/DBP, as well as its reciprocal) has been advanced as suitable candidates to evaluate hypertension and associated risks (Kerkhof *et al.*, 2022b). Concerning ratio-based approaches it was demonstrated that the fractional systolic (SBP/MAP) and diastolic (DBP/MAP) pressures are estimates of aortic pulsatility. Furthermore, the product of SBP and DBP matches the total peripheral resistance times the cardiac power product (Chemla *et al.*, 2005).

Not surprisingly, epidemiologists discovered that inclusion of MAP in cardiovascular risk analysis studies significantly adds incremental prognostic value to the exclusive use of PP (Selvaraj *et al.*, 2016; Haider *et al.*, 2003; Motau *et al.*, 2018). The explanation for this finding follows from the appreciation that the initial data pair {SBP, DBP} is mathematically equivalent to the combination of the two derived variables, here represented as PP and MAP. Thus, there exists no meaningful route to simplify matters, and attempts to rely on a single derived metric inevitably imply loss of information. This warning particularly applies to ratios where the physical dimension cancels out in the division, as is also the case for SBP/DBP, mentioned above. If yet for some reason preference is given to the analysis of the ratio, then a supplementary metric must be considered. Transformation of a primary data pair to their ratio in fact implies transition to a polar coordinate system, where the distance (calculated as the hypotenuse) reflects the second coordinate, existing besides the slope (or angle) which corresponds with the ratio (Fig. 1). We call this complementary component the "companion" to the

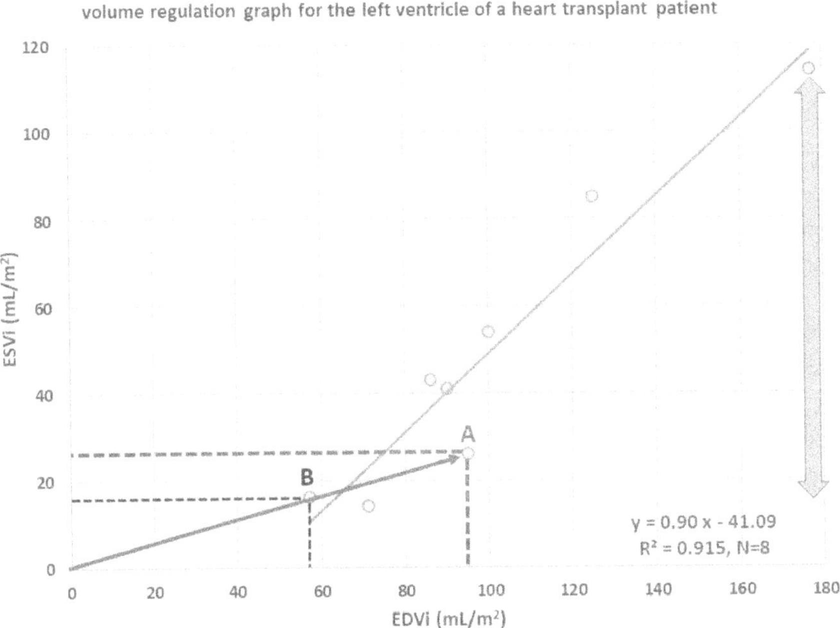

Fig. 1.   (Color online) ESVi versus EDVi for eight data pairs obtained by angiocardiography in a heart transplant patient over a period spanning more than 15 years. The entire collection yields a highly significant linear regression coefficient. The slope of 0.90 indicates that variation of EDVi is followed *pari passu* by values for ESVi. As the intercept on the abscissa is about 45 mL/m², while the slope is close to unity, it follows that the range for ESVi is wider than for EDVi, if expressed as percentage when upper limit is compared with lower limit. The yellow shaded area marks the territory from lowest ESVi to highest ESVi, showing an eight-fold range (from 14 to 114 mL/m², as indicated by the yellow arrowed bar), as opposed to a three-fold (i.e. 177/57 mL/m²) range for EDVi. Clearly, the slope of the line connecting individual data pairs with the origin at {0, 0} (see, for example, the red line with arrowhead) may differ widely for the various working points. This latter slope actually refers to polar coordinates. While the slope for points A and B is almost identical, their distance from the origin (being the second polar coordinate) differs. Based on data presented elsewhere (Kerkhof and Heyndrickx, 2021).

derived (ratio-based) metric. A major advantage of considering the companion obviously refers to the fact that it carries a sound physical dimension, in contrast to the ratio which is not unique and actually just a bare number.

Although featuring a physical dimension, a difference such as PP is not unique either, and therefore requires a companion, too. Mathematically seen, the derived metrics PP and SBP/DBP share the same companion (Kerkhof *et al.*, 2019b,e).

In this survey, we address ratio-based issues encountered in the evaluation of cardiac pump function on the basis of volume determination, besides a discussion of arterial blood pressure measurements, and evaluation of flow in the coronary system. For each situation, we demonstrate the need to consider the companion metric in addition to the use of a ratio or the difference as they are derived from primary data sets.

2. Introduction to Ventricular Performance Analysis

Ventricular function has been described by various approaches including pressure (P)–volume relationships with associated diastolic and systolic elastance curves, within the volume domain yielding unitless strain parameters, besides the working point concept and the dimensionless ejection fraction (EF), as well as time (t) derived indices such as dP/dt or circumferential fiber shortening velocity. Generally, all of them can be classified into one of two categories: those carrying physical dimensions and those that do not. The latter category is acceptable if accompanied by the associated complementary metric, but unfortunately this requirement has seldom been met. Failure to consider the companion which is inherently connected to ratio-based metrics has hampered progress in cardiophysiology for more than six decades. Various investigators admit that relying on EF alone provides an incomplete description (Manisty and Francis, 2008). Alternative routes have been indicated, partly referring to various types of strain measurements. However, most alternatives again concern dimensionless ratios leading to a perpetuation of the vague situation (Kerkhof and Handly, 2023). Recently, it was stated that in heart failure (HF) patients, EF should be supplemented or even replaced by more specific indices of left ventricle (LV) function such as the systolic strain, cardiac power output and size such as the LV diastolic diameters and volumes (Triposkiadis *et al.*, 2022). In fact, this formulation emphasizes the need to expand analysis by adding a variable to the traditional "monolith" EF. Technically seen, this notion is similar to the documented need in hemodynamics to analyze PP in conjunction with the surrogate MAP, as described above.

This contribution focuses on the exploration of the companion metric as applied to various ratio-based indexes used in cardiology. In contrast to the classical ratio-based metrics, all companions do carry physical units. This step forward may in particular induce a landslide in the traditional EF-based strategy to phenotype (or rather "ratiotype") HF subgroups. Based on a comprehensive description we start presenting a balanced survey on cardiac pump function that captures basic ventricular dynamics, energetic considerations, as well as clinically relevant corresponding prognostic outcomes. Next, we address aspects of arterial blood pressure, followed by a comprehensive evaluation of hemodynamics in the coronary circulation.

3. The Volume Domain Representation of Ventricular Mechanics

The heart has often been typified as a biological compression pump. This concept means that the dynamics of each of the four compartments can be described as a function of pressure (P), volume (V) and time (t). The LV is the major pumping chamber, generating the highest pressure level, compared to the right ventricle (RV) or either of the atria. Cavity volume may vary over a wide operating range, even during baseline conditions, and particularly with severe cardiopathology. As the operating range for LV volume may increase up to seven-fold during serious cardiac disease, it is attractive to consider LV volume as a primary characteristic of pump performance. In contrast, the systolic pressure level only varies by a factor of 2, implying that indeed LV volume is the dominant component in terms of disease-related variation. This notion led to the volume domain characterization of ventricular pump function, established by relating end-systolic volume (ESV) to end-diastolic volume (EDV), and resulting in the volume regulation graph (VRG). Figure 1 documents in the VRG representation the distribution of various volume data sets collected in a single patient following heart transplant (Kerkhof and Heyndrickx, 2021). Volumes have often been indexed (i) for body surface area, yielding end-systolic volume index (ESVi) and end-diastolic volume index (EDVi), expressed as mL/m^2. Each of these volume-based data pairs {EDVi, ESVi} defines an individual *working point*, i.e. the primary characteristics of the prevailing operating conditions (Kerkhof *et al.*, 2018a):

(1) the specific value for ESVi (which is important as it is associated with myocardial oxygen consumption);
(2) the filling volume EDVi (which along with ESVi determines the stroke volume index (SVi), and also cardiac output when combined with details on heart rate);
(3) a quantity that refers to stroke work (when details on systolic pressure are available);

(4) the {EDVi, ESVi} pair determines the location and roughly also the shape of the pressure–volume loop (again, when information on systolic pressure is available, which may be indirectly obtained, e.g. by noninvasively measuring brachial artery pressure).

The most pronounced variation is seen for ESVi (in Fig. 1, see yellow arrow, connecting the lowest with the highest ESVi value found). The broad range observed makes this variable an attractive candidate to evaluate ventricular function (Kerkhof *et al.*, 2018a). Parenthetically, this view indirectly supports a widely acclaimed clinical viewpoint stating that the popular metric termed EF is an appealing candidate to judge cardiac deterioration and evaluate ventricular response to treatment. Although EF is defined by the combination of ESVi and EDVi (namely by considering their ratio), it has been shown that actually ESVi is by far the most dominant determinant of EF (Kerkhof *et al.*, 2018d). Apart from considering the just mentioned ratio, recent attention has also been directed to the sum of ESVi and EDVi. This composite component has been incorporated into the global function index (GFI), which has been advanced as a superior alternative for EF, but has been seriously questioned elsewhere (Diaz-Navarro and Kerkhof, 2021).

It is well known that various reference values concerning variables and metrics (significantly) differ for men compared to women (Kerkhof *et al.*, 2018b). In this survey, we will not specifically address this important issue, as our principal emphasis is directed to comprehensive analysis strategies for data routinely measured in the clinical setting.

4. Coordinate System Transformation

The VRG representation based on ESVi (ordinate) and EDVi (abscissa) refers to the traditional Cartesian coordinate system. From a graphical point of view, the prevailing value for EF of each working point can be directly obtained from the VRG presentation by considering the slope of the line that connects the working point with the origin of the Cartesian coordinate system. The resulting value for EF, expressed as a fraction, equals (1-slope) (Faes and Kerkhof, 2015). Actually, the angle of this line reflects one of the two applicable *polar coordinates*. Note that EF is just a number, without physical dimensions, and its calculation is prone to measurement errors (Kerkhof *et al.*, 2022a). The associated second polar coordinate can be calculated as the distance from the origin to the working point under consideration, using the Pythagorean theorem for the hypotenuse (Kerkhof *et al.*, 2018c). As any hypotenuse is coupled to the prevailing EF in each working point, we have termed this particular volume the *companion* (C) of EF (denoted as EFC, expressed in mL, and mL/m^2 for EFCi). We have shown that EFC is associated with EDVi (Kerkhof *et al.*, 2019e). Obviously, both coordinate systems are equivalent in terms of information provided (Kerkhof *et al.*, 2022a).

The high linear correlation (typically R^2 is ≥ 0.80 for $N = 155$) found for ESVi and EDVi in cardiac patients means that their difference is fairly constant when the slope is close to unity (Kerkhof *et al.*, 2018d). This difference is termed SVi, and based on the regression equation yields $41.1 + 0.1$ EDVi (mL/m^2) in our example (Fig. 1). As EF is defined as SVi/EDVi, it follows that EF depends on the prevailing EDVi in numerator and denominator. Figure 1 illustrates that two (or more) working points can have the same value for EF, but distinct values for each associated EFC. Combining details on the polar coordinates, i.e. slope (as reflected by EF) and EFC permits an alternative description of any working point in the VRG.

The regression line shown in Fig. 1 deserves special attention, as the high correlation found suggests that this equation can be employed to more or less "delineate" the trajectory for working points in an individual patient. The temporal pattern of these data has been described in detail elsewhere (Kerkhof and Heyndrickx, 2021). It is important to point out that the slope of this regression line on the VRG is unrelated to the various slopes obtained in the polar coordinate description mentioned before (and in Fig. 1 illustrated by the blue and red line, respectively) (Faes and Kerkhof, 2015).

The equation for the regression line can also be employed to explore relationships with derived metrics such as EF. The primary variables ESV and EDV yield

$$\text{ESV} = \alpha + \beta \text{EDV}. \tag{1}$$

We derived an analytical expression by combining Eq. (1) with the definition formula for EF (here expressed as a fraction, not as a percentage):

$$\text{EF} = 1 + \gamma\{\text{ESV}/(\delta - \text{ESV})\} \tag{2}$$

with $\gamma = \beta/R^2$ and $\delta = \alpha - \text{EDV}_{\text{ave}}(1 - R^2)\beta/R^2$ where R^2 is the variance in ESV explained by the regression model in Eq. (1), while EDV_{ave} is the average value of EDV for the population under consideration. As expected, $\text{EF} = 1$ for $\text{ESV} = 0$, while the formula also captures the asymptotic range for higher ESV values (Fig. 2). This expression is more robust than the convenient logarithmic approach which generally fails to comply with the former two boundary conditions (Kerkhof *et al.*, 2018d).

In conclusion, we found that the primary variables involved in ventricular volume regulation in a single patient yield a fairly linear relationship

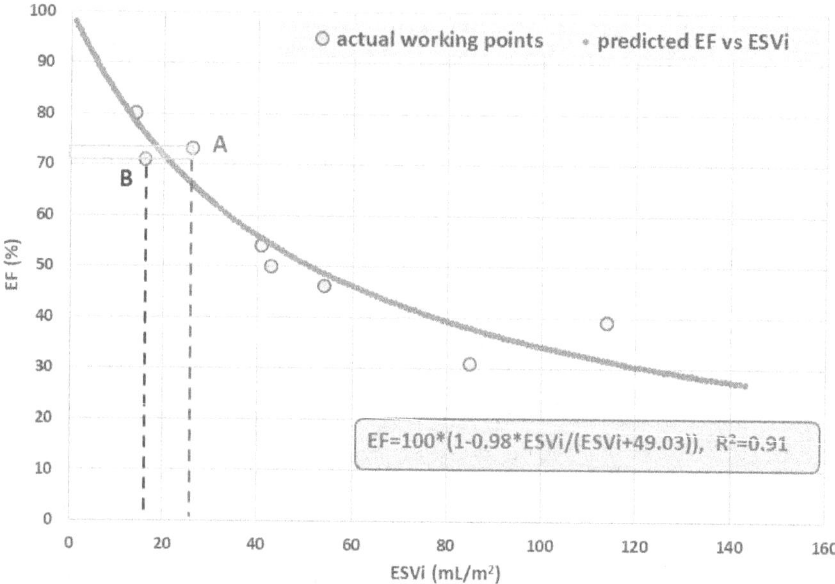

Fig. 2.   (Color online) EF (%) versus ESVi for the LV as angiocardiographically determined in the same patient as shown in Fig. 1. The high correlation coefficient for the predicted fit suggests a simple inverse association between the ratio-based metric EF and its principal component ESVi. The curve refers to the robust expression (Eq. (2)), as documented elsewhere (Kerkhof *et al.*, 2018d). Points A and B refer to two working points with nearly identical values for EF (indicated by the yellow bar), but distinguished by their differing ESVi measurement results. Obviously, in the asymptotic range (i.e. the part of the brown curve to the right) the ESVi becomes even more discriminative as the values for EF tend to level off.

(Kerkhof and Heyndrickx, 2021). The VRG representation based on these fundamental variables permits insightful visualization of the derived ratio-based metric EF (Beringer and Kerkhof, 1998), as well as its companion EFC (Kerkhof *et al.*, 2018c). Also, the association between the clinically frequently applied index EF and the key variable ESV can be formulated in an analytical expression.

5. Population-Based Studies: Healthy Individuals

In the previous section, we presented data on a single patient. However, the VRG approach can also be applied to a cohort of healthy individuals with a normal heart (Kerkhof *et al.*, 2018a), or to cardiac patients with either identical or distinct diagnoses referring to underlying cardiopathology (Kerkhof, 2016). Such a presentation consists of a superposition of individual {EDV, ESV} data pairs obtained from members within a group. Findings for 410 healthy adults (215 women) have been described elsewhere (Kerkhof *et al.*, 2018b). For linear regression in the VRG the $R^2 = 0.73$, and for EF versus ESVi the $R^2 = 0.30$ using a logarithmic approach. The latter value is rather low due to the fact that healthy persons tend to have very similar values for both ESVi and EDVi, which implies that the data points are located within a somewhat confined circular area within the VRG. Interestingly, EF values for healthy persons are around 62% (Mihaileanu and Antohi, 2020), as also observed for healthy adult mammals (Li, 1996), covering a range from rat to horse (Kerkhof *et al.*, 2019e). In contrast, there is a much lower correlation between EF and EDVi (Kerkhof *et al.*, 2018d). As EDV is the larger component in the expression for the hypotenuse, it is plausible to expect a strong correlation between the Cartesian coordinate EDVi and the associated EFCi (Kerkhof *et al.*, 2019e). The characteristic value of 62% for EF as often found in normal adults may not apply to all development states. For the mouse embryo, for example, we confirmed the familiar VRG (Fig. 3) but found 21 < EF < 40%, based on data published by

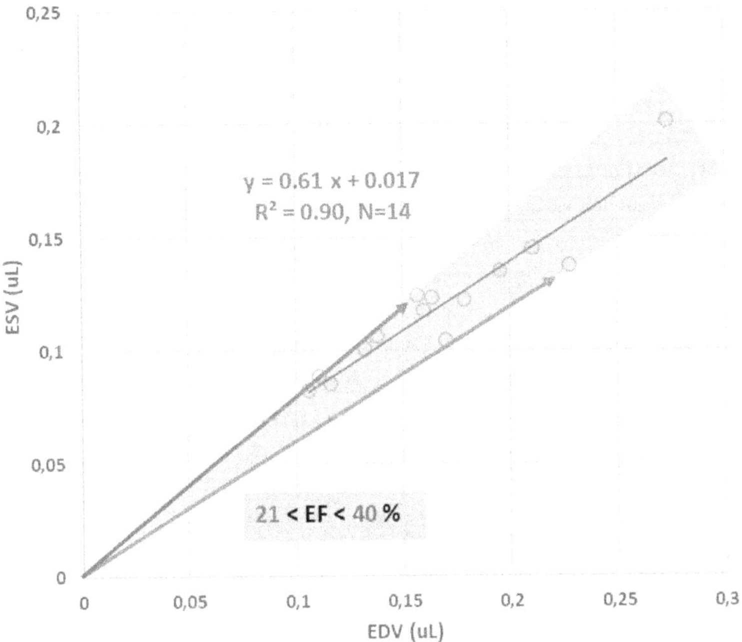

Fig. 3.   (Color online) Left ventricular volume determined in mice embryo (stage day 10.5) using intravital microscopy by transillumination as studied by Tanaka *et al.* (1997) permits derivation of the VRG and yields an excellent correlation for ESV versus EDV. The full range found for EF is marked by the gray triangular area, and refers to lower values than those obtained in healthy adult mammals. The minimal value for EF is 21% (green arrow) and the maximum 40% (blue arrow).

Tanaka *et al.* (1997). The low range for EF suggests that EF and ESV are somewhat uncoupled during this embryonal phase, possibly reflecting the asymptotic range (shown to the right in Fig. 2), or due to incomplete neural regulation of these developing hearts (Kerkhof *et al.*, 1981).

The VRG framework has been successfully applied in other studies (Uemura *et al.*, 2016; Mohammed *et al.*, 2021; Høilund-Carlsen *et al.*, 1988). Interestingly, it has also been found that during upright bicycle exercise in healthy human volunteers the ESV "follows" *pari passu* the EDV (Renlund *et al.*, 1990), suggesting that during physical activity similar patterns are present as those observed at baseline in healthy individuals (Kerkhof *et al.*, 2018a).

In summary, we found a linear relationship for LV ESVi versus EDVi of healthy individuals. The VRG offers a useful framework to introduce the polar coordinates EF and EFC(i), (Kerkhof *et al.*, 2018b).

6. Population-Based Studies: Cardiac Patients

Regarding patients with cardiac disease, we studied HF and various acute cardiac diseases. Heart disease is often accompanied by dilatation, possibly resulting in remodeling. For the VRG this means that the range of ESVi and EDVi values is extended compared to healthy individuals. As SVi remains fairly constant, this means that the values calculated for EF are deemed to decrease while the dilatation process progresses. Indeed, generally, a lower value for EF corresponds with poorer ventricular function as illustrated in Fig. 4 for 420 HF patients, evaluated by biplane angiocardiography. First, note that the volume ranges covered in these cardiac patients is much larger than the ones found for the "normals", with ESVi between 12.1 and 35.8 mL/m^2 for men ($N = 195$) and ESVi for women between 8.5 and 32.7 mL/m^2 ($N = 215$) according to echocardiography data as published elsewhere (Kerkhof *et al.*, 2018a). Second, various derived metrics such as SVi, EF and EFC can be visualized within the same framework. For example, in the VRG representation iso-EF lines can be constructed (such as the red one for EF = 75%). Additionally, iso-SV and iso-EFC trajectories can be inscribed (Kerkhof *et al.*, 2019e), providing insight into the consequences of variation of each parameter (Fig. 5). Note that values for SVi increase when going further down from the identity line (i.e. where ESVi = EDVi). The gray area in Fig. 4 indicates all working points with SVi < 50 mL/m^2, similar to those explored in a recent publication (Shah *et al.*, 2022). Combined with the requirement for supranormal EF (i.e. above 75%), this yields the small triangular area enclosed by the green lines.

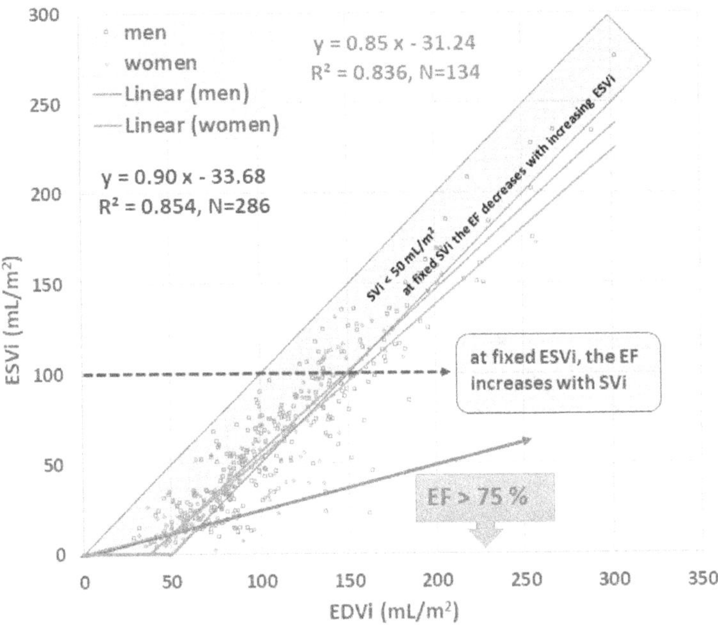

Fig. 4. (Color online) VRG for 420 HF patients, evaluated by angiography. The individual working point is indicated by the data pair of ESVi and EDVi. Regression lines for men and women are shown, along with the regression equations. The difference between EDVi and ESVi equals SVi. Working points located within the gray colored zone all have SVi < 50 mL/m². EF can be derived from the slope of the line obtained by connecting a working point with the origin {0, 0}. The red line with arrowhead indicates the trajectory where all points have EF = 75%. The area below this line covers all data points with supranormal EF, i.e. EF > 75%. Combining the requirements of EF > 75% and SVi < 50 mL/m² (as proposed by Shah *et al.* (2022)) yields the triangular area contained within the green lines, mostly including patients (69% women) with extremely small ESVi and EDVi values.

As healthy individuals are often found to have an EF around 62%, a value far above that level does not refer to something like an "even better than normal" heart. Indeed, a supranormal value for EF is a bad sign, as these extremely small hearts have a disproportionally high myocardial oxygen consumption (MVO_2) relative to the external work performed (Kerkhof *et al.*, 2018a; Kerkhof and Handly, 2020). Shah *et al.* (2022) found that prognosis is particularly poor for patients combining EF > 75% with small SVi. Figure 4 marks the region that meets these requirements, and illustrates the small ESVi values found for these patients. The optimum range for ESVi (Fig. 6) in terms of MVO_2 (Beringer and Kerkhof, 1998; Kerkhof *et al.*, 2018a; Kerkhof and Handly, 2020) can be "translated" into a similar optimum range for EF, while keeping in mind the relatively tight association between EF and ESVi (Fig. 2). Using machine learning it has been shown that

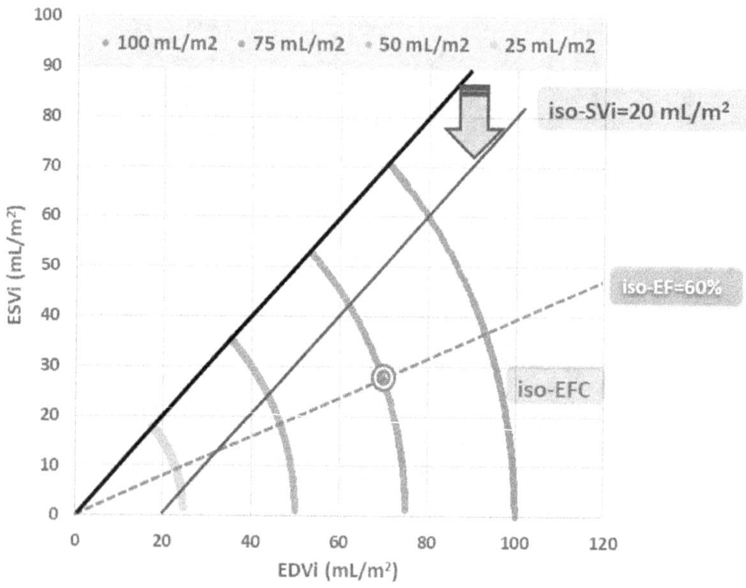

Fig. 5.   (Color online) Schematic VRG, relating ESVi to EDVi, while showing a trajectory for constant (iso-) EF, SVi and four curves for the EF companion (EFC). Considering a particular working point, such as the one marked by the red dot, this representation facilitates evaluating the joint consequences for ESVi, EDVi, SVi, EF and EFC when traversing the volume domain. Black line is the identity line, where ESVi = EDVi.

a cut-off value for ESVi set at 35 mL/m^2 can distinguish HFpEF patients from those with reduced EF (Alonso-Betanzos *et al.*, 2015), suggesting that a single variable with physical dimensions can readily replace the traditional ratiotyping approach. This finding has been further developed in a clinical study documenting the supremacy of ESVi over EF when classifying HF patients (Kerkhof *et al.*, 2019a; Kato *et al.*, 2020).

Traditionally, HF phenotypes have been based on particular ranges for EF, e.g. above 50% where EF is considered to be preserved. There is a tendency to split up the HF spectrum into strata of EF, implying that the impact of EFC becomes increasingly important for identifying working points once a particular "EF band" phenotype is selected. For example, the mid-range (mr) covers HF patients with 40% < EF < 50%. That definition refers to a range just half the size shown in Fig. 3, and therefore emphasizes the importance of EFC in these situations. Failure to recognize the impact of EFC may lead to confusion, and a few investigators have justly indicated that classification of HF phenotypes requires more than a single criterion based on EF (Boulet *et al.*, 2021). More specifically, we have proposed to explore a classification system principally based on ESV along with focus on sex-specific aspects (Kerkhof *et al.*, 2019a).

Recently, a HFpEF cohort was subdivided into two groups with 50% < EF < 60% and those with EF > 60%; not surprisingly distinct differences were found in terms of hypercontractile state and ventricular–arterial coupling (VAC) (Rosch *et al.*, 2022). As the current practice of HF phenotyping is solely based on cut-off values for the unitless metric EF, it would be better to employ the term "ratiotyping" for this dimensionless strategy.

In conclusion, the VRG framework displays the distribution of working points, and a wider range is observed for ESVi and EDVi in patients compared to healthy individuals. This volume domain representation also provides trajectories for situations with constant values for EF, EFC(i) and SV(i). Traditional ratiotyping (i.e. structured by EF-based stratification) of HF patients emphasizes the necessity to include EFC in order to attain a comprehensive evaluation.

7. Right Ventricle and Both Atria

The VRG for the LV yields highly significant linear correlations for an individual patient (Fig. 1), as well as for a cohort (Fig. 4). Similar results are obtained for the RV as reported elsewhere (Kerkhof *et al.*, 2018d). An example is presented here (Fig. 6). Comparable findings for the same patients were obtained for left and right atria ($N = 86$), with linear correlations of 0.88 and 0.86, respectively (Kerkhof *et al.*, 2022c).

8. Insights from the Volume Regulation Graph

The volume domain representation (Figs. 1, 3, 4 and 6) shows individual working points and permits derivation of a simple expression (Eq. (1)) to relate ESV(i) to EDV(i) for each cardiac compartment. This fundamental equation has been employed to model the association between EF and ESV (Eq. (2)), and even to predict myocardial oxygen consumption (MVO_2) as a function of ESV (Beringer and Kerkhof, 1998). Interestingly, the VRG concept appears applicable to both individual patients, as well as to cohort studies. The linear regression coefficients obtained from relating ESVi to EDVi permit reasonable prediction of interpolated data points, as well as derivation of analytical expressions that reliably describe the relationships between various derived metrics and the primary variables ESV and EDV. Previously we have shown that MVO_2 is associated with ESVi resembling a "swoosh"-shaped pattern, and for adult humans showing a nadir around a value of 20 mL/m^2 (Fig. 7). For values of ESVi below this point it

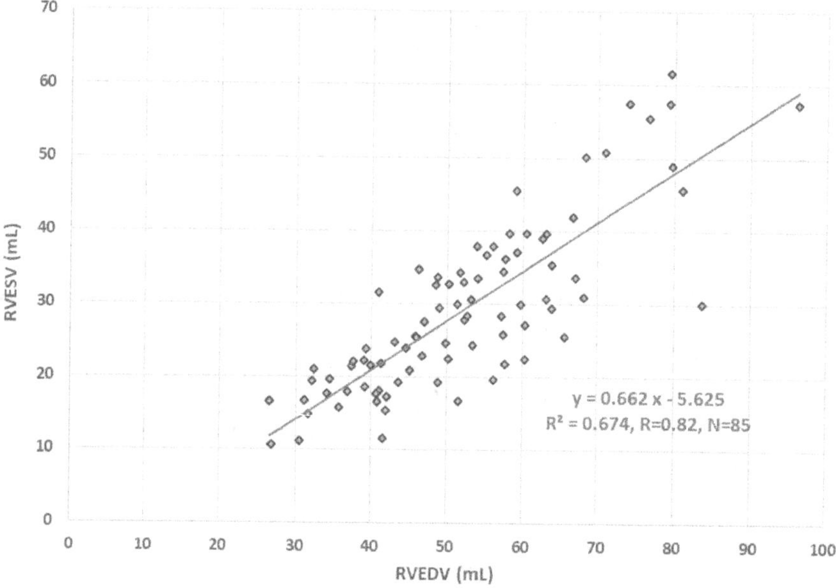

Fig. 6.   VRG for the RV volumes measured by cardiac magnetic resonance imaging, and showing 85 patients diagnosed with acute myocarditis ($N = 11$), acute myocardial infarction ($N = 59$), or takotsubo ($N = 15$). ESV, end-systolic volume; EDV, end-diastolic volume. Data made available by Prof. R. A. Diaz-Navarro (Valparaiso, Chile) (Diaz-Navarro and Kerkhof, 2021).

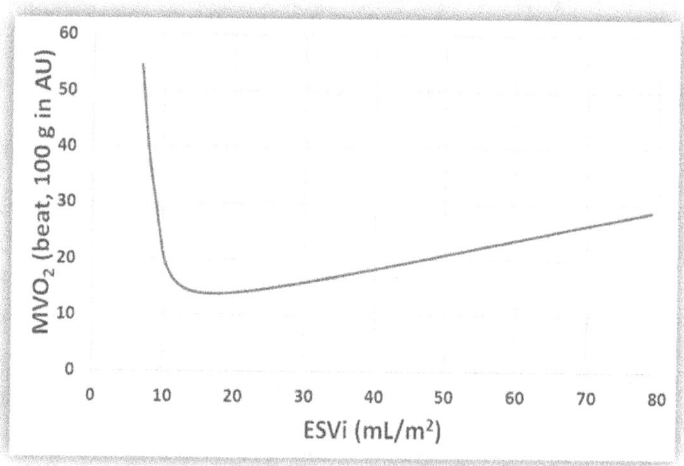

Fig. 7.   Schematic summary of the association between myocardial oxygen consumption (MVO_2) and ESVi. Note the nadir around 10 to 20 mL/m². AU means arbitrary units (Kerkhof *et al.*, 2018a).

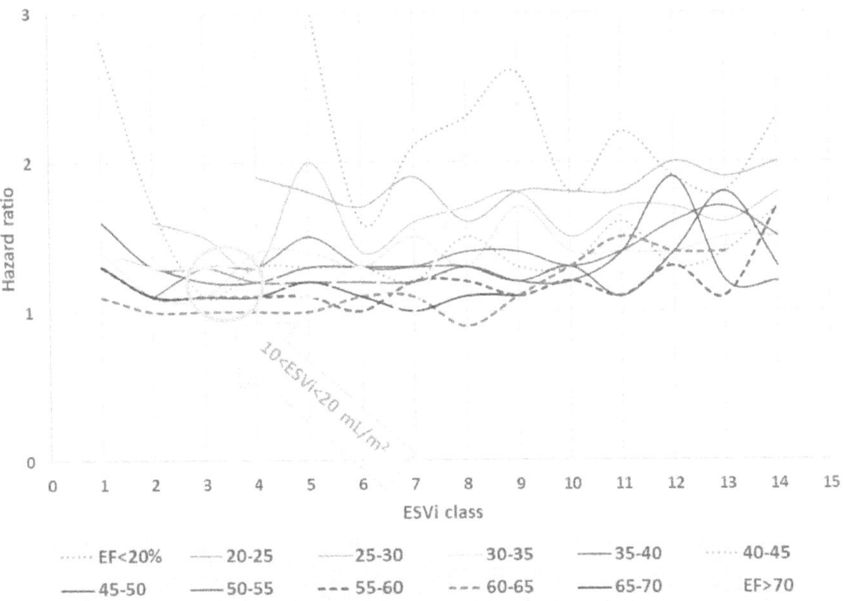

Fig. 8. (Color online) Adjusted hazard ratio (HR) for mortality versus ESVi at various levels of EF as specified in the gray colored box (N = 203,627). ESVi classes (bins) range from <5 and up to >65 mL/m^2 with steps of 5 mL/m^2. The yellow circular area marks the nadir for HR occurring for 10 < ESVi < 20 mL/m^2, and whose position applies to nearly all EF levels studied. Excluding ESVi classes 6 and 7, the EF range around the *sectio aurea* (i.e. 62%, see brown broken curve) steadily offers the lowest HR values up to class 9 (where 40 < EF < 45 mL/m^2 for ESVi). Data derived from Fig. S7A in Wehner *et al.* (2020).

can be seen that MVO$_2$ rises sharply, which observation readily explains why mortality dramatically increases for smaller ventricles (Kerkhof and Handly, 2020).

Supporting evidence for this concept can be derived from data by Curtis *et al.* using various imaging modalities (Curtis *et al.*, 2003), later confirmed by echocardiography data presented by Wehner *et al.* (2020). In Fig. 8, we show the adjusted hazard ratio versus ESVi for mortality as reported in their study. Clearly, for 10 < ESVi < 20 mL/m^2 all curves corresponding with various well-defined incremental EF ranges converge to the same low value for the hazard ratio (which refers to an effect size measure for time-to-event data). This nadir applies to most values of EF. For very low EF values an LV with a small ESVi simply cannot pump sufficient blood to perfuse all tissues. When EF = 25% and ESVi = 20 mL/m^2 (i.e. near the nadir), the SVi would be only 7 mL/m^2, generating a cardiac output of less than one L/min·m^2, even at a heart rate as high as 140 beats per minute, which pumping state is insufficient in an adult.

Interestingly, for 60% < EF < 65% the ratio remains low until ESVi > 45 mL/m^2, suggesting that the *sectio aurea* for EF-values occupies a preferred position (Mihaileanu and Antohi, 2020; Kerkhof *et al.*, 2019e). In an earlier study, Samad *et al.* (2019) found that addition of the component EF to machine learning-based multivariable approaches aiming to predict survival only modestly improved the performance across 10 models analyzed. A similar, but now sex-specific, study was reported by Stewart *et al.* (2021). Among patients investigated for suspected or established cardiovascular disease, these authors found clinically relevant sex-based differences in the distribution. Specifically, their data suggest a greater risk of mortality at higher EF levels among women.

The derived metric EF is a composite of two primary variables, namely ESV and EDV. Once focusing on ESVi it appears that there is only a minor role for EF to characterize ventricular function. This finding is not surprising when appreciating the paramount importance of minimizing MVO_2 and the connection with an optimal range for the primary variable ESVi (Fig. 4) which in turn points to the same narrow range for ESVi which corresponds with the lowest hazard ratio for mortality (Fig. 8). This comprehensive view unifies energetic, mechanical and prognostic aspects. Other studies have also highlighted the key role of ESV, for example in relation to diastolic recoil (Kato *et al.*, 2020).

An independent study by Stewart *et al.* confirms that mortality is highest for EF < 40%, and these authors also point out distinct age-related risk patterns for men and women (Stewart *et al.*, 2021).

9. VRG and Pressure–Volume Loop

Thus far, we discussed primary variables and derived metrics referring to ventricular volumes only. However, to more adequately describe cardiac pumping action it is required to include ventricular pressure data, and describe the time-dependent trajectory in the pressure–volume domain (Fig. 9). The contours and especially the location of the loops are very characteristic when control and depressed situation are compared. Although pressure levels may vary to some extent, it is clear that ESVi is the main determinant, given that SVi spans a well-defined range as modulated by heart rate (Kerkhof *et al.*, 2018a). Therefore, the pressure–volume loop largely reflects the working point as defined by {EDVi, ESVi}, as introduced above.

Apart from the primary variables that refer to pressure and volume, we may also consider derived metrics, including two types of elastances and notably their ratio which became very popular. End-systolic elastance (Ees) refers to the ratio

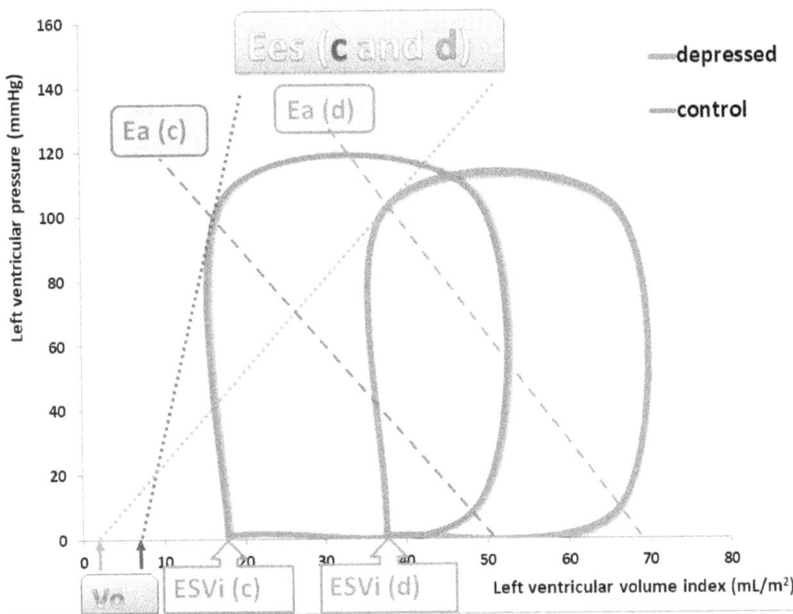

Fig. 9.   (Color online) Schematic presentation of pressure–volume loops for the LV, referring to the control (*c*) and depressed (*d*) state, respectively. ESVi plays a central role, not only by defining the end-contraction volume for each loop, but also by being an essential determinant of end-systolic elastance (Ees) and effective arterial elastance (Ea). The intercepts Vo (see purple and blue arrows) correspond with the Ees slopes for the *c* and *d* states, respectively.

of pressure and volume, both considered at end-systole. For successive data points this line does not automatically cross the origin of the coordinate system, but rather leaves an abscissal intercept (Vo) which may be small or large (and even negative) (Kerkhof *et al.*, 2022d; Antohi *et al.*, 2022). Effective arterial elastance (Ea) is defined as the ratio of pressure at the same moment, divided by SVi. To return to the simplicity of dimensionless metrics, the VAC index is defined as Ees/Ea or as its reciprocal. Thus, VAC = SVi/(ESVi-Vo), which reduces to a trivial variant of EF if Vo is assumed to be zero (Kerkhof *et al.*, 2018a). Note that the dimensionless number calculated for VAC does not depend on pressure, as it merely refers to the ratio of volumes. Thus, all efforts invested in obtaining a more comprehensive description by including pressure have been eliminated by relying on VAC if indeed Vo is neglected. Recently, a more advanced route has been proposed by not only considering pressure and volume, but also by introducing time intervals (Antohi *et al.*, 2022).

10. Companion Metrics: A Broader View

We have emphasized the need to consider a companion whenever considering a dimensionless ratio-based metric such as EF. As candidate EFC we have proposed the hypotenuse that can be calculated using the Pythagorean theorem. However, the hypotenuse is just one obvious candidate for choosing a companion associated with a difference-based or ratio-based metric (Kerkhof *et al.*, 2019e). In fact, any well-defined mathematical construct that is founded on the two primary variables can do the job. The calculation of the hypotenuse refers to the quadratic mean, and differs only by a constant multiplier, namely $1/(\sqrt{2}) = 0.71$ which term originates from the definition for quadratic mean: $\sqrt{\{(a^2 + b^2)/2\}}$ (Fig. 10). Besides the quadratic mean (or hypotenuse) we may also consider arithmetic, harmonic or geometric means. Their graphical definitions are shown in Fig. 10. The arithmetic mean, defined as (EDVi + ESVi)/2 is already applied in a new index to evaluate LV function, namely the GFI as recently critically analyzed (Diaz-Navarro and Kerkhof, 2021). Furthermore, we have the geometric mean $M = \sqrt{(a \times b)}$ and the harmonic mean $H = 2 \times (a \times b)/(a + b)$. Of course, one may think of other choices (such as $\{a\sqrt{b}\}$ or $\{b^2\sqrt{a}\}$) which all will be applicable as long as they are uniquely defined. The attractive goal is of course to develop a construct that has meaningful affinity with any physiologically relevant properties. For example, the derived metric *mean arterial blood pressure* (and being a surrogate of the PP companion) is a sound candidate in hemodynamics as it connects mean flow to blood vessel resistance (Kerkhof *et al.*, 2019e).

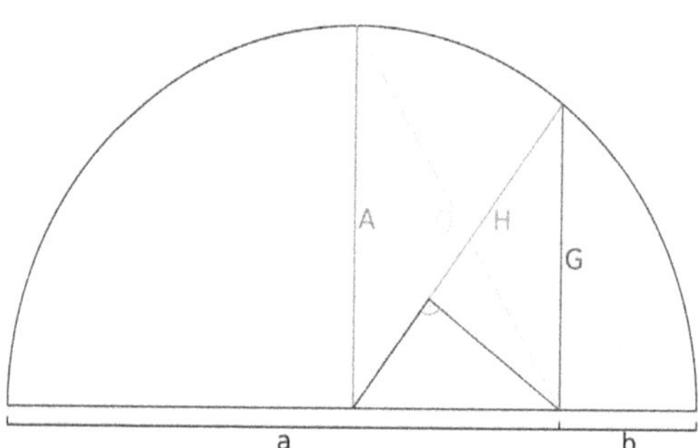

Fig. 10.   Various Pythagorean means as alternative candidates for the hypotenuse as companion metric. The line segments *a* and *b* can be incorporated into appropriate formulas to yield the arithmetic (*A*), geometric (*G*), harmonic (*H*) or quadratic (*Q*) mean. Figure taken from https://en.wikipedia.org/wiki/Pythagorean_means. See also Pythagorean means — from Wolfram MathWorld.

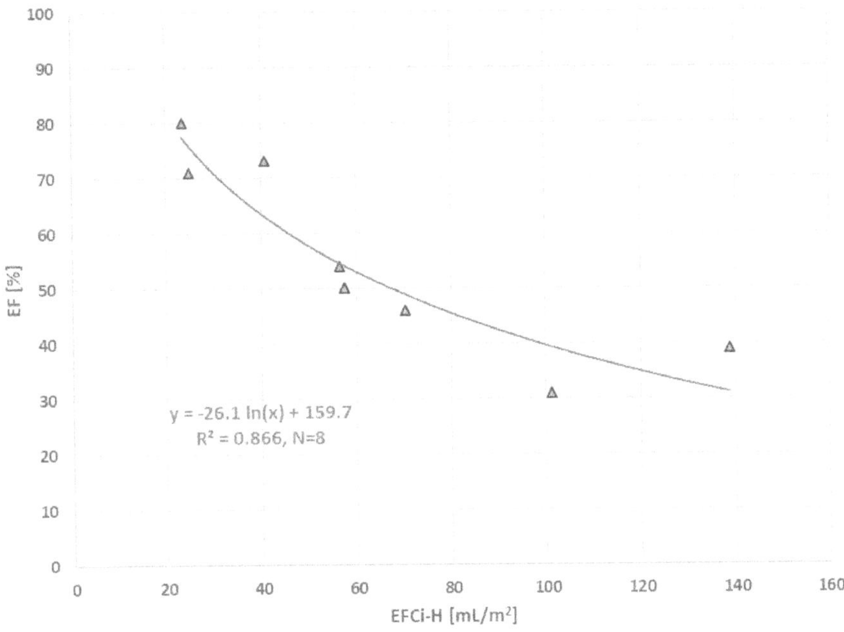

Fig. 11. Selecting the harmonic (H) variant of the indexed (i) EF companion (EFCi-H) of the Pythagorean means as the companion metric associated with EF, yields a highly significant logarithmic relationship with EF. Same patient data as in Fig. 1. Based on data presented elsewhere (Kerkhof and Heyndrickx, 2021).

As an example, the harmonic (H) version of a companion to EF is presented in Fig. 11. This EFCi-H is defined as 2/{1/ESVi + 1/EDVi)}, and can be compared with the hypotenuse variant as shown in Fig. 1).

11. Applications in the Field of Arterial Blood Pressure

Hemodynamics concerns the study of pressure, flow and resistance (or impedance when considering phasic phenomena). Resistance refers to mean values for pressure and flow, as expressed in the Poiseuille formula for laminar flow and a given pressure gradient (Li, 2000). MAP is often calculated as 1/3 of the sum of SBP and twice the value recorded for the DBP.

Guidelines on the interpretation of arterial blood pressure levels are still a matter of intense debate. Discussion initially concentrated on the relative importance of SBP and DBP. Later MAP was also considered a relevant metric, while epidemiologists pointed to the impact of PP, being the difference between SBP and DBP. Even the ratio of SBP and DBP found wide applications, e.g. in the calculation of pulse wave velocity (Avolio *et al.*, 2018; Li, 2000), or the estimation of Ees (Antohi *et al.*, 2022).

A problem, not often recognized, arises from the fact that a difference such as PP is not uniquely defined (Kerkhof *et al.*, 2019b), and suffers from the same shortcomings as the corresponding ratio-based metric. Thus, consideration of a companion metric is required (Kerkhof *et al.*, 2019b). This subject has been elaborated on by Konradi cs., and extended to the augmentation index (Konradi *et al.*, 2020). It was found that PPC (i.e. the companion to PP) is nicely correlated with MAP, thus illustrating that PP and MAP form a logical tandem. In fact, MAP may be viewed as a surrogate for the mandatory PPC. Interestingly, pieces of the blood pressure puzzle further come together by the observation that the ratio of SBP and DBP is associated with the value calculated for their difference (which is PP) (Kerkhof *et al.*, 2022b). Figure 12 illustrates the inverse association between two derived metrics (here the ratio and the difference of arterial blood pressure), referring to the primary SBP and DBP.

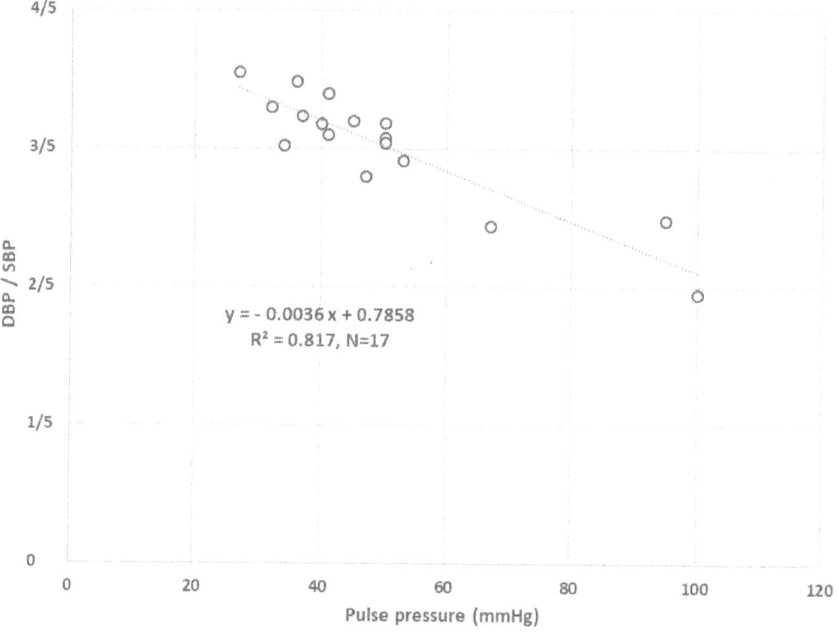

Fig. 12. Inverse linear relationship between two derived metrics, namely the ratio and the difference of paired primary variables, here referring to arterial DBP and SBP. Data points concern the same patients as in Fig. 6 (women only). Based on Kerkhof *et al.* (2022b).

Another derived metric concerns the augmentation index (AIx), defined as augmentation pressure divided by PP (Avolio *et al.*, 2018). Application of the companion concept to AIx has been described by Fukuie *et al.* (2021a,b). Furthermore, the dimensionless index (DI) is a useful parameter to express the size of the effective valvular area as a proportion of the cross-section area of the LV outflow tract (OT) velocity-time integral (VTI) to that of the aortic valve jet, and is calculated by the ratio of the subvalvular velocity obtained by pulsed-wave Doppler (LVOT-VTI) divided by the maximum velocity measured by continuous-wave Doppler across the aortic valve (AV-VTI). The impact of the DI companion was studied in patients with severe aortic stenosis (Mantha *et al.*, 2021).

12. Applications in the Evaluation of Coronary Flow

The central subject in the study of the coronary circulation concerns delivery of adequate blood flow to the myocardium, which amounts up to 10% of the total pumped out by the LV. Limited coronary flow, e.g. due to epicardial arterial stenosis, may give rise to severe cardiac problems, possibly even resulting in death. Measurement of flow at baseline and during induced hyperemia permits calculation of their ratio, called coronary flow reserve (CFR). Again, comprehensive interpretation of this ratio requires consideration of the associated companion (CFRC) (Cecere *et al.*, 2022; Tona *et al.*, 2022).

As measurement of local pressure in an artery is technically more feasible, an alternative route has been developed to estimate severity of an occlusion. During hyperemia, post-stenotic mean pressure is measured in combination with mean aortic pressure. Their ratio is termed fractional flow reserve (FFR) with a cut-off value at 0.80 to guide the decision about intervention. To complement this dimensionless metric we introduced the FFR companion (denoted as FFRC) (Kerkhof *et al.*, 2019d).

Pressure-based efforts were initiated when in earlier times it was determined that visual inspection of the stenosis (using angiocardiography) is inadequate to determine the extent of the stenosis. It was theoretically derived that a sigmoid association exists for FFR and percentage of cross-sectional area stenosis (Faes *et al.*, 2020). Figure 13 shows FFR versus the stenotic pressure gradient for patients with varying degrees of coronary artery stenosis, illustrating the association between two derived metrics.

Table 1 summarizes the various primary variables discussed in this review, along with their main derived metrics and companions.

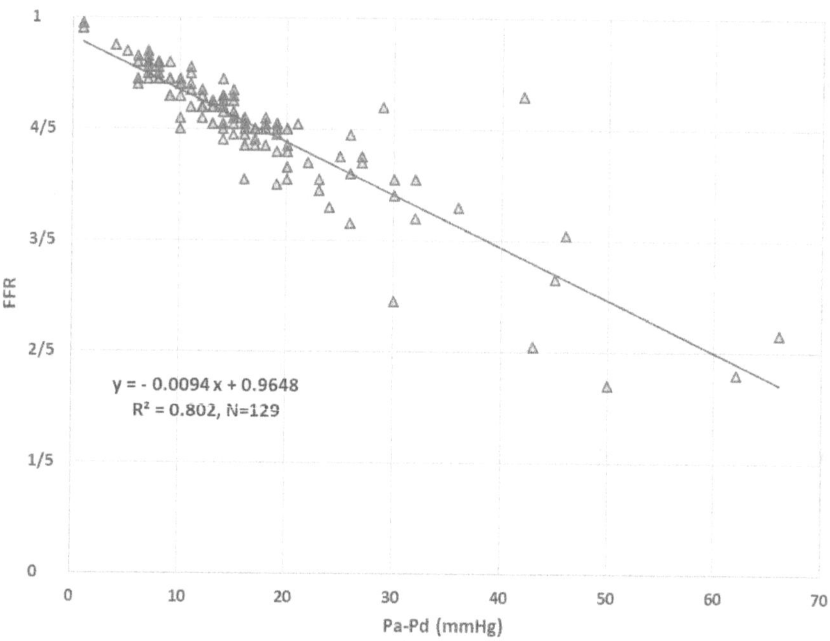

Fig. 13.   Inverse linear relationship between two derived metrics, namely the ratio and the difference of paired primary variables, here referring to mean aortic pressure (Pa) and mean post-stenotic coronary artery pressure (Pd), both obtained during hyperemia in 129 patients with (partial) coronary artery occlusion. Modified from Kerkhof *et al.* (2019d).

Table 1.   Summary of primary variables and derived metrics for four application areas as discussed in this survey. Each companion is calculated by applying the Pythagorean theorem to the two primary variables. Acronyms: DPVr, diastolic peak velocity at rest; DPVh, diastolic peak velocity during hyperemia; other acronyms as defined in the main text.

	Primary	Derived	Companion
Ventricular volume	ESV(i)	SV(i)	EFC
	EDV(i)	EF	EFC
Arterial blood pressure	DBP	PP	PPC
	SBP	DBP/SBP	PPC
	PP	AIx	AIxC
	AP		
Coronary pressure	Pd	FFR	FFRC
	Pa		
Coronary flow	DPVr	CFR	CFRC
	DPVh		

13. Conclusions

Cardiovascular investigations often concern paired measurements that provide the primary variables. From these basic data additional metrics have been derived, mainly referring to differences or ratios. As those derived metrics are not unique when used in isolation, we propose inclusion of associated companion metrics in order to offer a comprehensive analysis. The idea of introducing a companion fills the gap that is created by combining two measurement data into a single number obtained by taking their ratio or difference. Of course, there is a wide choice for defining such a companion. In this study, we explored Pythagorean means as candidates. That approach differs from the procedure applied to normalization of data, where the new metric becomes dimensionless, in contrast to the companions we introduced.

References

Alonso-Betanzos, A, Bolón-Canedo, V, Heyndrickx, GR and Kerkhof, PL (2015) Exploring guidelines for classification of major heart failure subtypes by using machine learning, *Clin. Med. Insights Cardiol.* **9** (Suppl 1), 57–71, doi:10.4137/CMC.S18746.

Antohi, EL, Chioncel, O and Mihaileanu, S (2022) Overcoming the limits of ejection fraction and ventricular–arterial coupling in heart failure, *Front. Cardiovasc. Med.* **8**, 750965, doi:10.3389/fcvm.2021.750965.

Avolio, AP, Kuznetsova, T, Heyndrickx, GR, Kerkhof, PLM and Li, J-KJ (2018) Arterial flow, pulse pressure and pulse wave velocity in men and women at various ages, *Adv. Exp. Med. Biol.* **1065**, 153–168, doi:10.1007/978-3-319-77932-4_10.

Beringer, JY and Kerkhof, PL (1998) A unifying representation of ventricular volumetric indexes, *IEEE Trans. Biomed. Eng.* **45**(3), 365–371, doi:10.1109/10.661161.

Boulet, J, Massie, E and Rouleau, JL (2021) Heart failure with midrange ejection fraction — What is it, if anything? *Can. J. Cardiol.* **37**(4), 585–594, doi:10.1016/j.cjca.2020.11.013.

Cecere, A, Kerkhof, PLM, Civieri, G, Angelini, A, Gambino, A, Fraiese, A, Bottio, T, Osto, E, Famoso, G, Fedrigo, M, Giacomin, E, Toscano, G, Montisci, R, Iliceto, S, Gerosa, G and Tona, F (2022) Coronary flow evaluation in heart transplant patients compared to healthy controls documents the superiority of coronary flow velocity reserve companion as diagnostic and prognostic tool, *Front. Cardiovasc. Med.* **9**, 887370, doi:10.3389/fcvm.2022.887370.

Chemla, D, Antony, I, Zamani, K and Nitenberg, A (2005) Mean aortic pressure is the geometric mean of systolic and diastolic aortic pressure in resting humans, *J. Appl. Physiol.* **99**(6), 2278–2284, doi:10.1152/japplphysiol.00713.2005.

Curtis, JP, Sokol, SI, Wang, Y, Rathore, SS, Ko, DT, Jadbabaie, F, Portnay, EL, Marshalko, SJ, Radford, MJ and Krumholz, HM (2003) The association of left ventricular ejection fraction, mortality, and cause of death in stable outpatients with heart failure, *J. Am. Coll. Cardiol.* **42**(4), 736–742, doi:10.1016/s0735-1097(03)00789-7.

Diaz-Navarro, RA and Kerkhof, PLM (2021) Left ventricular global function index and the impact of its companion metric, *Front. Cardiovasc. Med.* **8**, 695883, doi:10.3389/fcvm.2021.695883.

Faes, TJ and Kerkhof, PL (2015) The volume regulation graph versus the ejection fraction as metrics of left ventricular performance in heart failure with and without a preserved ejection fraction: A mathematical model study, *Clin. Med. Insights Cardiol.* **9** (Suppl 1), 73–91, doi:10.4137/CMC.S18748.

Faes, TJC, Meer, R, Heyndrickx, GR and Kerkhof, PLM (2020) Fractional flow reserve evaluated as metric of coronary stenosis — A mathematical model study, *Front. Cardiovasc. Med.* **6**, 189, doi:10.3389/fcvm.2019.00189.

Fukuie, M, Hoshi, D, Hashitomi, T, Watanabe, K, Tarumi, T and Sugawara, J (2021a) Exercise in water provides better cardiac energy efficiency than on land, *Front. Cardiovasc. Med.* **8**, 747841, doi:10.3389/fcvm.2021.747841.

Fukuie, M, Yamabe, T, Hoshi, D, Hashitomi, T, Nomura, Y and Sugawara J (2021b) Effect of aquatic exercise training on aortic hemodynamics in middle-aged and elderly adults, *Front. Cardiovasc. Med.* **8**, 770519, doi:10.3389/fcvm.2021.770519.

Haider, AW, Larson, MG, Franklin, SS and Levy, D (2003) Systolic blood pressure, diastolic blood pressure, and pulse pressure as predictors of risk for congestive heart failure in the Framingham Heart Study, *Ann. Intern. Med.* **138**(1), 10–16.

Høilund-Carlsen, PF *et al.* (1988) The reliability of measuring left ventricular ejection fraction by radionuclide cardiography: Evaluation by the method of variance components, *Br. Heart J.* **59**(6), 653–662, doi:10.1136/hrt.59.6.653.

Kato, M, Kitada, S, Kawada, Y, Nakasuka, K, Kikuchi, S, Seo, Y and Ohte, N (2020) Left ventricular end-systolic volume is a reliable predictor of new-onset heart failure with preserved left ventricular ejection fraction, *Cardiol. Res. Pract.* **2020**, 3106012, doi:10.1155/2020/3106012.

Kerkhof, PL (2016) Fundamentals of left ventricular volume representation, in *2016 38th Annual Int Conf IEEE Engineering in Medicine and Biology Society* (*EMBC*) (IEEE), pp. 3294–3297, doi:10.1109/EMBC.2016.7591432.

Kerkhof, PL, Baan, J, Buis, B and Arntzenius, AC (1981) Relations between ejection fraction and ventricular volume, and their alteration by chronic beta-blockade, *Br. Heart J.* **46**(1), 17–22, doi:10.1136/hrt.46.1.17.

Kerkhof, PLM, Diaz-Navarro, RA, Heyndrickx, GR and Handly, N (2022a) La serendipia en torno a la fracción de eyección: Una revisión de la historia, la casualidad y la cuasi-funcionalidad de una métrica aplaudida, *Rev. Med. Chile* **150**(2), 232–240, doi:10.4067/S0034-98872022000200232.

Kerkhof, PLM, Diaz-Navarro, RA, Heyndrickx, GR, Konradi, AO, Shlyakhto, EV, Handly, N and Li, JK (2022b) The ratio of diastolic and systolic arterial pressure is associated with pulse pressure, in *2022 44th Annual Int Conf IEEE Engineering in Medicine & Biology Society* (*EMBC*) (IEEE), pp. 1–4, doi:10.1109/EMBC48229.2022.9871478.

Kerkhof, PLM and Fu, Q (2022) Editorial: Fundamental enrichment of ratio-based metrics in cardiology, *Front. Cardiovasc. Med.* **9**, 1013194, doi:10.3389/fcvm.2022.1013194.

Kerkhof, PLM and Handly, N (2020) Insights from physiology applied to interpretation of supranormal ejection fraction in women, *Eur. Heart J. Cardiovasc. Imaging* **21**(4), 375–377, doi:10.1093/ ehjci/jeaa018.

Kerkhof, PLM and Handly, N (2023) In search for the optimal ventricular systolic dysfunction metric that associates with reduced exercise capacity, *J. Clin. Ultrasound* **51**(1), 16–19, doi:10.1002/ JCU.23262.

Kerkhof, PLM and Heyndrickx, GR (2021) Case report on the importance of longitudinal analysis of left ventricular end-systolic volume, rather than ejection fraction, in a heart transplant patient, *Eur. Heart J. Case Rep.* **5**(6), ytab146, doi:10.1093/ehjcr/ytab146.

Kerkhof, PLM, Heyndrickx, GR, Diaz-Navarro, RA, Antohi, EL, Mihaileanu, S and Handly N (2022c) Ventricular and atrial ejection fractions are associated with mean compartmental cavity volume in cardiac disease, in *2022 44th Annual Int Conf IEEE Engineering in Medicine & Biology Society* (*EMBC*) (IEEE), pp. 1384–1387, doi:10.1109/EMBC48229.2022.9871315.

Kerkhof, PLM, Heyndrickx, GR and Handly, N (2019a) Heart failure phenotypes require sex-specific criteria which are based on ventricular dimensions, in *2019 41st Annual Int Conf IEEE Engineering in Medicine and Biology Society* (*EMBC*) (IEEE), pp. 4909–4912, doi:10.1109/ EMBC.2019.8857165.

Kerkhof, PLM, Konradi, AO, Shlyakhto, EV, Handly, N and Li, J-KJ (2019b) Polar coordinate description of blood pressure measurements and implications for sex-specific and personalized analysis, in *2019 41st Annual Int Conf IEEE Engineering in Medicine and Biology Society* (*EMBC*) (IEEE), pp. 502–505, doi:10.1109/EMBC.2019.8857346.

Kerkhof, PLM, Kuznetsova, T, Ali, R and Handly, N (2018a) Left ventricular volume analysis as a basic tool to describe cardiac function, *Adv. Physiol. Educ.* **42**(1), 130–139, doi:10.1152/ advan.00140.2017.

Kerkhof, PLM, Kuznetsova, T, Kresh, JY and Handly, N (2018b) Cardiophysiology illustrated by comparing ventricular volumes in healthy adult males and females, *Adv. Exp. Med. Biol.* **1065**, 123–138, doi:10.1007/978-3-319-77932-4_8.

Kerkhof, PLM, Li, JK and Handly, N (2019c) Interpretation of a new biomarker for the right ventricle introduced to evaluate the severity of pulmonary arterial hypertension, *Pulm. Circ.* **9**(2), 2045894019826945, doi:10.1177/2045894019826945.

Kerkhof, PLM, Li, JK and Handly, N (2022d) Various approaches to define the volume intercept of the ventricular end-systolic pressure–volume relationship: Implications for statistical analysis, in *2022 44th Annual Int Conf IEEE Engineering in Medicine & Biology Society* (*EMBC*) (IEEE), pp. 1398–1401, doi:10.1109/EMBC48229.2022.9871671.

Kerkhof, PLM, Mérillon, JP, Yoo, BW, Peace, RA, Parry, G, Heyndrickx, GR, Kuznetsova, T, Meijboom, LJ, Sprengers, RW, Park, HK and Handly, N (2018c) The Pythagorean theorem reveals the inherent companion of cardiac ejection fraction, *Int. J. Cardiol.* **270**, 237–243, doi:10.1016/j.ijcard.2018.06.074.

Kerkhof, PLM and Miller, VM (eds.) (2018) *Sex-Specific Analysis of Cardiovascular Function* (Springer, Cham), ISBN-10: 3319779311.

Kerkhof, PLM, Osto, E, Tona, F, Heyndrickx, GR and Handly, N (2019d) Sex-specific interpretation of coronary flow reserve and fractional flow reserve metrics, including their companions, in *2019 41st Annual Int Conf IEEE Engineering in Medicine and Biology Society* (*EMBC*) (IEEE), pp. 7006–7009, doi:10.1109/EMBC.2019.8857589.

Kerkhof, PLM, Peace, RA and Handly, N (2019e) Ratiology and a complementary class of metrics for cardiovascular investigations, *Physiology* (*Bethesda*) **34**(4), 250–263, doi:10.1152/ physiol.00056.2018.

Kerkhof, PLM, van de Ven, PM, Yoo, B, Peace, RA, Heyndrickx, GR and Handly, N (2018d) Ejection fraction as related to basic components in the left and right ventricular volume domains, *Int. J. Cardiol.* **255**, 105–110, doi:10.1016/j.ijcard.2017.09.019.

Konradi, AO, Maslyansky, AL, Kolesova, E, Shlyakhto, EV and Kerkhof, PLM (2020) Role of ratio-based metrics in cardiology, *Russ. J. Cardiol.* **25**(10), 3929.

Li, JK-J (1996) *Comparative Cardiovascular Dynamics of Mammals* (CRC Press, Boca Raton, FL).

Li JK-J (2000) *The Arterial Circulation: Physical Principles and Clinical Applications* (Humana Press, Totowa, NJ).

Manisty, CH and Francis, DP (2008) Ejection fraction: A measure of desperation? *Heart* **94**(4), 400–401, doi:10.1136/hrt.2007.118976.

Mantha, Y, Futami, S, Moriyama, S and Hieda, M (2021) Valvulo-arterial impedance and dimensionless index for risk stratifying patients with severe aortic stenosis, *Front. Cardiovasc. Med.* **8**, 742297, doi:10.3389/fcvm.2021.742297.

Mihaileanu, S and Antohi, EL (2020) Revisiting the relationship between left ventricular ejection fraction and ventricular–arterial coupling, *ESC Heart Fail.* **7**(5), 2214–2222, doi:10.1002/ ehf2.12880.

Mohammed, H, El-Feshawy, M, Basiony, F and Abu shady, M (2021) Role of lung ultrasound and inferior vena cava diameter in assessment of patients with heart failure, *Egypt. J. Hosp. Med.* **85**(2), 4102–4107, doi:10.21608/ejhm.2021.207097.

Motau, TH, Norton, GR, Sareli, P and Woodiwiss, AJ (2018) Aortic pulse pressure does not adequately index cardiovascular risk factor-related changes in aortic stiffness and forward wave pressure, *Am. J. Hypertens.* **31**(9), 981–987, doi:10.1093/ajh/hpy061.

Renlund, DG, Gerstenblith, G, Fleg, JL, Becker, LC and Lakatta, EG (1990) Interaction between left ventricular end-diastolic and end-systolic volumes in normal humans, *Am. J. Physiol.* **258** (2 Pt 2), H473–H481, doi:10.1152/ajpheart.1990.258.2.H473.

Rosch, S, Kresoja, KP, Besler, C, Fengler, K, Schöber, AR, von Roeder, M, Lücke, C, Gutberlet, M, Klingel, K, Thiele, H, Rommel, KP and Lurz, P (2022) Characteristics of heart failure with preserved ejection fraction across the range of left ventricular ejection fraction, *Circulation* **146**(7), 506–518, doi:10.1161/CIRCULATIONAHA.122.059280.

Samad, MD, Ulloa, A, Wehner, GJ, Jing, L, Hartzel, D, Good, CW, Williams, BA, Haggerty, CM and Fornwalt, BK (2019) Predicting survival from large echocardiography and electronic health record datasets: Optimization with machine learning, *JACC Cardiovasc. Imaging* **12**(4), 681–689, doi:10.1016/j.jcmg.2018.04.026.

Selvaraj, S, Steg, PG, Elbez, Y, Sorbets, E, Feldman, LJ, Eagle, KA, Ohman, EM, Blacher, J, Bhatt, DL and REACH Registry Investigators (2016) Pulse pressure and risk for cardiovascular events in patients with atherothrombosis: From the REACH registry, *J. Am. Coll. Cardiol.* **67**(4), 392–403, doi:10.1016/j.jacc.2015.10.084.

Shah, S, Segar, MW, Kondamudi, N, Ayers, C, Chandra, A, Matulevicius, S, Agusala, K, Peshock, R, Abbara, S, Michos, ED, Drazner, MH, Lima, JAC, Longstreth Jr., WT and Pandey, A (2022) Supranormal left ventricular ejection fraction, stroke volume, and cardiovascular risk: findings from population-based cohort studies, *JACC Heart Fail.* **10**(8), 583–594, doi:10.1016/j.jchf.2022.05.007.

Stewart, S, Playford, D, Scalia, GM, Currie, P, Celermajer, DS, Prior, D, Codde, J, Strange, G and NEDA Investigators (2021) Ejection fraction and mortality: A nationwide register-based cohort study of 499 153 women and men, *Eur. J. Heart Fail.* **23**(3), 406–416, doi:10.1002/ejhf.2047.

Tanaka, N, Mao, L, DeLano, FA, Sentianin, EM, Chien, KR, Schmid-Schönbein, GW and Ross Jr., J (1997) Left ventricular volumes and function in the embryonic mouse heart, *Am. J. Physiol.* **273**(3 Pt 2), H1368–H1376, doi:10.1152/ajpheart.1997.273.3.H1368.

Tona, F, Osto, E, Kerkhof, PLM, Montisci, R, Famoso, G, Lorenzoni, G, De Michieli, L, Cecere, A, Zanetti, I, Civieri, G, Iliceto, S and Piaserico, S (2022) Multiparametric analysis of coronary flow in psoriasis using a coronary flow reserve companion, *Eur. J. Clin. Invest.* **52**(4), e13711, doi:10.1111/eci.13711.

Triposkiadis, F, Giamouzis, G, Kitai, T, Skoularigis, J, Starling, RC and Xanthopoulos, A (2022) A holistic view of advanced heart failure, *Life* (*Basel*) **12**(9), 1298, doi:10.3390/life12091298.

Uemura, K, Kawada, T, Zheng, C and Sugimachi, M (2016) Less invasive and inotrope-reduction approach to automated closed-loop control of hemodynamics in decompensated heart failure, *IEEE Trans. Biomed. Eng.* **63**(8), 1699–1708, doi:10.1109/TBME.2015.2499782.

Wehner, GJ, Jing, L, Haggerty, CM, Suever, JD, Leader, JB, Hartzel, DN, Kirchner, HL, Manus, JNA, James, N, Ayar, Z, Gladding, P, Good, CW, Cleland, JGF and Fornwalt, BK (2020) Routinely reported ejection fraction and mortality in clinical practice: Where does the nadir of risk lie? *Eur. Heart J.* **41**(12), 1249–1257, doi:10.1093/eurheartj/ehz550.

CHAPTER 4

Mathematical Model to Study the Squeeze Film Characteristics of Diseased Human Synovial Knee Joint[a]

Mo Sadique[*] and Sapna Ratan Shah[†]

*School of Computational & Integrative Sciences,
Jawaharlal Nehru University, India*
[*]Sadique93ms@gmail.com
[†]sapna1980jan@gmail.com

Synovial fluid functions as a biological lubricant and lubricates articular cartilage to reduce friction and wear. Lubricin and hyaluronic acid are the primary components of synovial fluid responsible for its lubricating properties. The loss of properties in synovial fluid and articular cartilage due to aging and activities can restrict mobility in synovial joints, resulting in the degradation of articular cartilage and ultimately leading to pathological synovial joints, which is a major cause of disability. Thus, research on synovial joints remains crucial, and despite previous investigations on synovial joint lubrication, there are several issues related to squeeze film lubrication that require further attention. The Newtonian model of squeeze film lubrication in synovial joints needs to be extensively studied. In this study, lubrication and other related properties of synovial fluid are studied theoretically. In this paper, we have studied the flow of synovial fluid in the diseased synovial joint. Further, we have studied the effect of the viscosity of the synovial fluid, the permeability of articular cartilage, thickness of articular cartilage, and fluid film thickness on the characteristic of the squeeze film formed between the articular cartilages of the diseased human knee joint. The flow of synovial fluid is modeled by considering it as a viscous, incompressible and Newtonian fluid. We have derived the modified Reynolds equation using the principle of hydrodynamic lubrication and continuum mechanics theory and solved it by applying the suitable boundary conditions according to the physical considerations. Subsequently, we obtained the expression for pressure distribution in fluid film, load-bearing capacity, and squeeze time and have done the theoretical analysis on these properties for different parameters. Pressure increases with squeeze velocity and viscosity of the synovial fluid and decreases with permeability and fluid film thickness. Human knee joint becomes diseased due to excessive pressure, and the mobility of the knee joint decreases. The load capacity

---

[*]Corresponding author.
[a]This article was previously published in *World Scientific Annual Review of Biomechanics*. Vol: 1, (2023) 2330004 (21 pages).

increases with viscosity and squeeze velocity and decreases with permeability resulting in the reduction of the load-carrying capacity of the knee joint in diseased conditions. Moreover, the squeeze time also increased in the diseased state of the joint.

Keywords: Synovial fluid; Reynolds equation; hyaluronic acid; squeeze films; Brinkman equation; arthritis.

1. Introduction

Synovial joints are the most significant characteristic of the human body since they are the epicenter of the most basic and vital function in humans, which is mobility. A synovial joint is a load-bearing system composed of two mating bones that move in tangential and normal directions. A soft sponge-like material known as articular cartilage covers the end of the two mating bones. The joint space is filled with a shear-dependent fluid known as synovial fluid, which fills the space between these cartilaginous ends of the bones. The synovial fluid is a transparent yellowish dialysate of blood plasma with hyaluronic acid content. Synovial fluid provides lubrication to the synovial joint in order to reduce the wear and friction between the mating bones and articular cartilage during the motion. It enhances the mechanical functioning of the synovial joint. The thin coating of synovial fluid that covers the surfaces of the joint capsule's inner layer and articular cartilage serves to maintain the joint surfaces lubricated and minimizes friction. Pores of the articular cartilage are very small, and hyaluronic acid molecules do not typically pass through the pores of the articular cartilage (Bazrov, 2010; Kudenatti *et al.*, 2013).

Synovial fluid is a viscoelastic polymeric solution, Ogston and Stanier (1953) demonstrated this fact, and Gibbs *et al.* (1968) later confirmed it. They studied the effect of external stimulation on the viscoelastic properties of synovial fluid (Damiano and Bardin, 2004). Recently Mathieu *et al.* (2009) also suggested the non-Newtonian and viscoelastic nature of the synovial fluid. Despite strong evidence of synovial fluid being viscoelastic, there are a number of publications, which tells about the viscous nature of the synovial fluid (Naduvinamani and Savitramma, 2013; Kumar and Raghavendra, 2015; Kudenatti *et al.*, 2013). Synovial fluid behaves as viscous fluid as long as it is not under external stimulation. It is shown that the viscoelastic behavior of the synovial fluid depends on the concentration of the hyaluronic acid (Deheri *et al.*, 2011). The synovial fluid behaves as a non-Newtonian pseudoplastic fluid, and its viscosity is affected by the concentration of hyaluronic acid molecules present in it (Dintenfass, 1963). It is experimentally established that under certain physical considerations, synovial fluid is viscous-like and incompressible, and its viscosity depends on the shear rate and concentration of hyaluronan (Coffman, 1980;

Davies, 1966). The surface of the cartilage of a sick joint can become rough and fractured, and the permeability of articular cartilage increases due to pathological conditions. The hyaluronic acid molecules enter into cartilage, and the synovial fluid can lose its non-Newtonian behavior. In diseased conditions, synovial fluid loses its non-Newtonian behavior, and it becomes Newtonian (Hays, 1963). It is considered in this present work that the synovial fluid is a viscous, Newtonian, and incompressible fluid. There are number of inflammatory and degenerative conditions that affect synovial joints. Bursitis and tendonitis, as well as other kinds of arthritis and Lyme disease, are examples of inflammatory joint disorders. There are more than a hundred types of degenerative and inflammatory joint disorders referred to as arthritis. Chronic forms of arthritis include osteoarthritis, rheumatoid arthritis, and gouty arthritis.

The most prevalent kind of arthritis is osteoarthritis, which develops when the cartilage of the human synovial joint wears away. Osteoarthritis is the most common chronic form of arthritis. It is a chronic degenerative condition, often called wear-and-tear arthritis. The bone ends are exposed due to this, allowing them to grind together. Because of this issue, the synovial joint may have stiffness, discomfort, and loss of mobility. Osteoarthritis is a widespread illness that affects the load-bearing joints of the body, and it can be caused by a variety of factors, including trauma, heredity, obesity, and others. On the other hand, rheumatoid arthritis is a chronic autoimmune disease, and it starts with the swelling of the synovial membrane (Hays, 1963). Synovial fluid is supposed to behave as a lubricant along with its two other essential functions, providing nutrition to the cartilage and removing metabolite from it. Thus, synovial fluid behaves as a lubricant in synovial joints (Kudenatti *et al.*, 2013). Further, Kumar and Raghavendra (2015) discussed in detail about the lubricating properties of synovial fluid, and Dintenfass (1963) discussed the lubrication mechanism in synovial joints in different conditions, and he arrived at a conclusion about the presence of hydrodynamic and squeezed film lubrication in Synovial joints and Naduvinamani *et al.* (2004) further confirmed this fact. Scientists and mathematicians have conducted mathematical analyses of squeeze films on a number of occasions. This squeeze film examination covers a study of the pressure distribution and load-bearing capability of squeeze films, as well as the approaching times of the lubricating surfaces. Hays (1963) investigated the properties of squeeze films between parallel rectangular plates of finite and infinite length and compared the results for both cases. Shukla (1978) studied the squeeze films between parallel plates in which one is flat and the other with curvature and the effect of the curvature of the surface of plates on the formation of squeeze films. Wu (1972) investigated the squeeze films formed between parallel rectangular plates, one of which had a porous face.

Verschoor (1951) investigated the effect of the porous facing of the plates on squeeze films and discovered that the porosity of the plate has a substantial effect on the squeeze film characteristics. The synovial joint is lubricated by the synovial fluid, which is primarily composed of lubricin and hyaluronic acid. There are different types of lubrication mechanisms that occur in the synovial joint. These mechanisms involve a different process for each type of lubrication. The lubricin molecules adsorb onto the surface of the articular cartilage and form a protective layer that reduces friction between the opposing surfaces of the joint in the squeeze film lubrication. The synovial membrane plays a crucial role in the lubrication process by secreting synovial fluid, which contains lubricating molecules and provides nutrients to the articular cartilage. The synovial membrane behaves as a unidirectional valve, and the synovial fluid enters easily into the joint space without escaping from the space. Articular cartilage, on the other hand, is responsible for absorbing shock and distributing the load across the joint, which helps to maintain the joint's lubrication and overall health. Therefore, both the articular cartilage and synovial membrane play important roles in the lubrication of the synovial joint (Hui *et al.*, 2012; Ruggiero, 2020; Klein, 2006). Shukla (1978) developed a new theory for the lubrication of rough surfaces, derived a generalized form of the Reynolds equation, and studied the effect of surface roughness on squeeze films. It has been shown in the work that the load capacity increases when the roughness of the mating surfaces increases. Naduvinamani *et al.* (2004) presented a theoretical investigation of the combined impact of lubricant ingredients and the roughness of the surface on the characteristics of squeeze film between two rectangular plates of fixed dimensions by deriving stochastic Reynolds equation and assuming the lubricant as a couple stress Stokes fluid. Sinha *et al.* (1982) and Deheri *et al.* (2011) did a theoretical analysis of squeeze films between rough, porous rectangular plates and computed the pressure variation and load capacity of these squeeze films. Naduvinamani and Savitramma (2013) studied surface roughness and poroelasticity effect on squeeze films of micropolar fluid between rectangular plates and further referred this study to the synovial joint lubrication. The analysis of the effect of surface roughness on squeeze film was done in this study, and it was shown that surface roughness has a considerable effect on the lubrication mechanism of synovial joints. Kudenatti *et al.* (2013) numerically solved the MHD Reynolds equation for a squeeze film of couple-stress fluids and studied the characteristics and effect of surface roughness on this squeeze film. Recently, Kumar and Raghavendra (2015) theoretically analyzed the surface roughness effect on the squeeze film formed in spherical bearings based on the deterministic approach of hydrodynamic lubrication and further derived a generalized form of the Reynolds equation. Singh *et al.* (1988) studied the significance

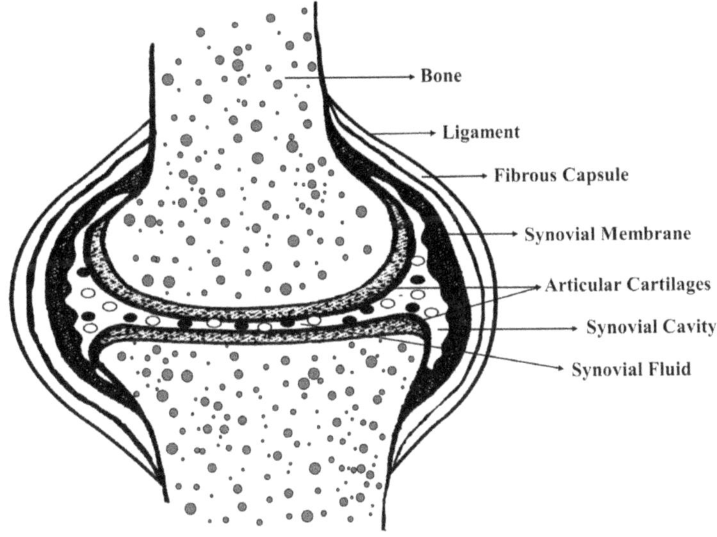

Fig. 1.   Synovial joint Sadique *et al.* (2023).

of squeeze film between parallel plates, and examined the surface roughness effect on this film. Figure 1 shows the schematic representation of the human synovial joint. In the present problem, we have studied the squeeze film formed in synovial joints and examined the significance of the properties of this squeeze film on the diagnosis of the disease related to synovial joints.

2. Mathematical Model

2.1. *Formulation of problem*

The flow of synovial fluid in diseased human knee joint under loading conditions has been considered in this work, which is based on the principles of lubrication theory and bio-fluid dynamics. Articular cartilage is considered as a porous material, and the length of the cartilage is much larger than the width to make the human knee joint geometry similar to the parallel plate model. The human knee joint is divided into two regions; the first one is the fluid film, and the second is the cartilage region. The symmetric case of the human knee joint has been considered for computing the velocity in both regions. Figure 2 represents the simple symmetrical geometry of the human knee joint, and Fig. 3 shows the parallel plate approximation of the human knee joint that we have considered for this study. The governing equations for the flow of synovial fluid in fluid film region

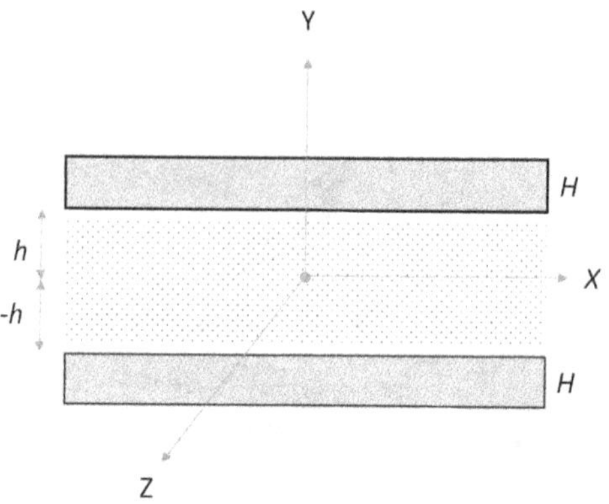

Fig. 2.   Simple geometry (symmetric case).

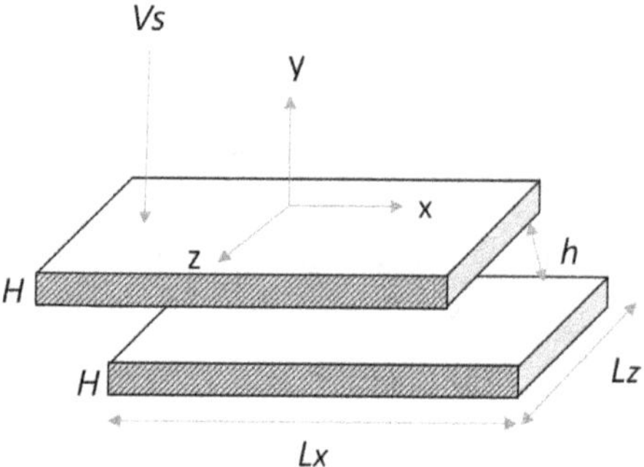

Fig. 3.   Parallel plate geometry of synovial joint.

are derived from the well-known Navier–Stokes equations for the flows of New-tonian fluids by imposing the restriction according to physical conditions. Darcy's law for flow in porous medium governs fluid flow in the porous medium. Synovial fluid flow in the cartilage region is governed by Brinkman's equation, which is an extension of Darcy's law (Verschoor, 1951). Further, the modified Reynolds equation is derived for the pressure variation in fluid film and cartilage regions, and load capacity and squeeze time are calculated for both regions. We have considered the synovial fluid as incompressible, non-conducting, and non-magnetic, and the flow of synovial fluid is laminar and steady; hence the variation of any property of synovial fluid with time is zero, and this flow is due to pressure gradient. The synovial fluid has been considered as an incompressible fluid since its density and volume remain constant irrespective of applied pressure due to its higher viscosity and high resistance to the flow. Therefore, we have assumed the synovial fluid as incompressible. The synovial fluid has also been assumed to be non-conducting as it is a very poor conductor of electricity due to the very few amounts of charged particles or ions in it. The non-magnetic nature of the synovial fluid is due to its low magnetic susceptibility. The synovial fluid behaves as a diamagnetic material due to its atomic and molecular structure. Since the diamagnetic materials are weakly repelled by the applied magnetic field and non-magnetic due to net zero magnetic moment, the synovial fluid can be assumed as non-magnetic.

The flow of synovial fluid is laminar and steady, and hence the variation of any property of synovial fluid with time is zero, and this flow is due to pressure gradient. In addition, we have considered the variation of pressure along fluid film thickness as zero.

Further, we have assumed that there are no external forces present, while gravitational forces are always present, but these forces are small enough so that their effect can be considered as negligible, and no-slip boundary conditions are assumed at the cartilage surfaces. The external forces have been considered negligible in this study since they are very small compared to the internal forces generated by the synovial joint itself. This is due to the fact that the synovial joint is surrounded by the ligaments, tendons, and other soft tissues providing resistance to external forces. By applying all these assumptions, Brinkman's equation and Navier–Stokes equation reduce into the following form, which governs the flow of synovial fluid in both the regions.

2.2. *Governing equations*

Region I: Fluid Film Region $0 \leq y \leq h$.

Navier–Stokes equations are a set of partial differential equations that describe the motion of fluid in space. These equations govern fluid flow and are used to predict the behavior of fluids, including the velocity, pressure, and density of the fluid at any given point in space and time. The Navier–Stokes equations provide a mathematical framework for understanding the behavior of the fluid flow.

The general form of the momentum balance and mass conservation equations of Navier–Stokes equations are given as follows:

$$\rho\left(\frac{\partial V}{\partial t} + V \cdot \nabla V\right) = -\nabla P + \mu \nabla^2 V + f.$$

Here, ρ is the density of the fluid, t is time, V is the velocity vector, P is the pressure, μ is the dynamic viscosity of the fluid, and f is the external force per unit mass acting on the fluid.

The conservation of mass is given by the continuity equation, and the general form of this equation is given as follows:

$$\frac{\partial \rho}{\partial t} + \frac{\partial}{\partial x}(\rho u) + \frac{\partial}{\partial x}(\rho v) + \frac{\partial}{\partial x}(\rho w) = 0.$$

Here u, v and w are the velocities of the fluid in x, y and z directions.

By applying the assumptions to the above momentum balance equation, we have obtained the following equations that govern the flow of synovial fluid. These equations are as follows:

$$\mu \frac{\partial^2 u_1}{\partial y^2} - \frac{\partial P}{\partial x} = 0,$$

$$\mu \frac{\partial^2 v_1}{\partial y^2} - \frac{\partial P}{\partial z} = 0, \tag{1}$$

$$\frac{\partial P}{\partial y} = 0.$$

Here u_1 and v_1 represent the velocity of the synovial fluid in the fluid film region, the symbol μ denotes the viscosity of the synovial fluid, P denotes the pressure distribution in synovial fluid film and articular cartilage. The symbols x, y and z denote the axial distances of Cartesian co-ordinates and these axial directions have been shown in Figs. 2 and 3.

Region II: Articular Cartilage Region $0 \leq y \leq h + H$.
The Brinkman equation is an attempt to explain the flow of fluid in a porous medium with non-zero velocity gradients, particularly at low Reynolds numbers. This equation modifies the conventional Darcy law by including a viscosity component with a coefficient that is typically associated with the viscosity of the fluid. The Brinkman equation is also referred to as the Darcy–Brinkman equation, and it serves as a governing equation for fluid flow through porous media that involves an additional Laplacian, known as the viscous or Brinkman factor. This equation has found extensive use in evaluating porous media with high porosity. The equation can be expressed as follows:

$$\mu' \frac{\partial^2 u_2}{\partial y^2} - \frac{\mu}{\varphi_1} u_2 - \frac{\partial P}{\partial x} = 0,$$

$$\mu' \frac{\partial^2 v_2}{\partial y^2} - \frac{\mu}{\varphi_2} v_2 - \frac{\partial P}{\partial z} = 0, \tag{2}$$

$$\frac{\partial P}{\partial y} = 0.$$

The above equations given by (2) have been derived from Darcy's law for fluid flows in the porous medium. These equations are the extended forms of Darcy's equation. These equations are utilized to determine the velocity of the synovial fluid in the articular cartilage of the synovial joint in axial directions. The velocity of the synovial fluid in articular cartilage in the x and z directions is represented by u_2 and v_2. The apparent viscosity of the synovial fluid is denoted by the symbol μ', while the permeability of the articular cartilage in the x and z directions is denoted by φ_1 and φ_2 respectively.

Additionally, symbol H represents the thickness of the articular cartilage, h denotes the thickness of the fluid film in the synovial cavity, and the symbols x, y and z in the equation represent the axial directions. The axial directions have been shown in Figs. 2 and 3.

2.3. *Boundary conditions and matching conditions*

The boundary condition for synovial fluid flowing in the fluid film region is given by

$$\frac{\partial u_1}{\partial y} = 0 \quad \text{at } y = 0 \quad \text{and} \quad \frac{\partial v_1}{\partial y} = 0 \quad \text{at } y = 0. \tag{3}$$

Boundary conditions for synovial fluid flowing in cartilage are given as follows:

$$u_2 = 0 \quad \text{at } y = h + H \quad \text{and} \quad v_2 = 0 \quad \text{at } y = h + H. \tag{4}$$

Considering our assumption of no-slip boundary condition, the velocity of the synovial fluid in the fluid film region and articular cartilage region at the interface, where cartilage meets with the fluid film region, must be the same. Therefore, the matching conditions for the velocities at the interface are as follows:

$$u_1 = u_2 = V_x \quad \text{and} \quad v_1 = v_2 = V_z \quad \text{at } y = h, \tag{5}$$

where V_x and V_z are the velocity of the synovial fluid at the interface in x and z directions, respectively. The layer of the synovial fluid and articular cartilage are two different phases of materials. The fluid film behaves as a fluid, and articular cartilage is a porous material. During the squeezing process, the synovial fluid flows into the articular cartilage, and a layer of synovial fluid is generated between the articular cartilage. A shear stress is present at this interface, which is parallel to the interface. This shear stress is caused due to the force exerted by the motion of the synovial fluid. This shear stress is tangential to the interface and must be equal for both synovial fluid and articular cartilage. If the shear stress is not equal at the interface, then there will be slippage or separation between the synovial fluid layer and articular cartilage. Since we have assumed the no-slip boundary condition at the interface, therefore the shear stresses at the interface must be equal for both regions.

Shear stresses at the interface are also the same. Therefore, we have the following matching condition for shear stresses:

$$\mu\frac{\partial^2 u_1}{\partial y^2} = \mu'\frac{\partial^2 v_1}{\partial y^2} \quad \text{and} \quad \mu\frac{\partial^2 u_2}{\partial y^2} = \mu'\frac{\partial^2 v_2}{\partial y^2} \quad \text{at } y = h. \tag{6}$$

Now we solve the equations governing the flow of synovial fluid in fluid film and articular cartilage given in Eqs. (1) and (2) with the help of boundary conditions and matching conditions given in Eqs. (3)–(5). By solving these equations, we find the velocity of synovial fluid in the fluid film region and articular cartilage.

The velocity of the synovial fluid in the fluid film region in both directions is obtained by solving Eq. (1) with the help of boundary conditions given in Eq. (3) and matching conditions given in Eq. (5). The velocities of synovial fluid in fluid film in the x and z directions are given as follows:

$$u_1 = \frac{1}{\mu}\frac{\partial P}{\partial x}(y^2 - h^2) + V_x,$$

$$v_1 = \frac{1}{\mu}\frac{\partial P}{\partial z}(y^2 - h^2) + V_z.$$

The velocity of synovial fluid in articular cartilage in both directions is obtained by solving Eq. (2) with the help of boundary conditions given in Eq. (4) and matching conditions given in Eq. (5). The velocities of synovial fluid in articular cartilage in the x and z directions are given as follows:

$$u_2 = \frac{\varphi_1}{\mu}\frac{\partial P}{\partial x}\frac{1}{\sinh(M_xH)}[\sinh M_x(h+H-y) - \sinh M_x(h-y)$$

$$- \sinh(M_xH)] + \left[\frac{V_x\sinh M_x(h+H-y)}{\sinh(M_xH)}\right],$$

$$v_2 = \frac{\varphi_2}{\mu}\frac{\partial P}{\partial z}\frac{1}{\sinh(M_zH)}[\sinh M_z(h+H-y) - \sinh M_z(h-y)$$

$$- \sinh(M_zH)] + \left[\frac{V_z\sinh M_z(h+H-y)}{\sinh(M_zH)}\right].$$

The symbols M_x and M_z are expressions involving some physical parameters, and we have written these symbols to represent the above velocity expression in a simplistic form. These symbols M_x and M_z are given as follows:

$$M_x = \left(\frac{\mu}{\mu' \varphi_1}\right)^{1/2},$$

$$M_z = \left(\frac{\mu}{\mu' \varphi_2}\right)^{1/2}.$$

The velocity at the interface, the region at which fluid film and articular cartilage meet with each other, can be found using the matching condition for shear stress given in Eq. (6).

The velocity of the synovial fluid at the interface is given by

$$V_x = \frac{\varphi_1}{\mu} \frac{\partial P}{\partial x} \tanh(M_x H)\left[\tanh\left(\frac{M_x H}{2}\right) - M_x h\right],$$

$$V_z = \frac{\varphi_2}{\mu} \frac{\partial P}{\partial z} \tanh(M_z H)\left[\tanh\left(\frac{M_z H}{2}\right) - M_z h\right].$$

The volumetric flow rate of a fluid is the amount of volume of the fluid passing through a surface per unit of time. This volumetric flow rate is calculated by integrating the velocity. Therefore, synovial fluid flux in both directions is calculated by the integration of velocity with respect to y, starting from the initial value as zero to a final value $(h + H)$. Synovial fluid fluxes Q_x and Q_z are calculated as follows:

$$Q_x = \int_0^h u_1 dy + \int_h^{h+H} u_2 dy.$$

Now putting the expressions of u_1 and u_2 in the above integral, we get the following:

$$Q_x = \int_0^h \left[\frac{1}{\mu}\frac{\partial P}{\partial x}(y^2 - h^2) + V_x\right]dy + \int_h^{h+H}\left[\frac{V_x \sinh M_x(h+H-y)}{\sinh(M_x H)}\right]dy + \int_h^{h+H}$$

$$\times \left[\frac{\varphi_1}{\mu}\frac{\partial P}{\partial x}\frac{1}{\sinh M_x H}(\sinh M_x(h+H-y) - \sinh M_x(h-y) - \sinh(M_x H))\right]dy.$$

By integrating the above integrals and simplifying the expressions, we get the expression for the synovial fluid flux in pathological synovial joint in the x-direction.

$$Q_x = -\frac{\partial P}{\partial x}\left[\frac{1}{M_x^3 \mu'}\left(\tanh M_x H\left(M_x h - \tanh\frac{M_x H}{2}\right)^2 + M_x H + 2\tanh\frac{M_x H}{2}\right) + \frac{h^3}{3\mu}\right].$$

$$(7)$$

Similarly, the volumetric synovial fluid flux in pathological synovial joint in the z-direction is calculated as follows:

$$Q_z = \int_0^h v_1 dy + \int_h^{h+H} v_2 dy.$$

Now putting the expressions of v_1 and v_2 in the above integral, we get the following:

$$Q_z = \int_0^h \left[\frac{1}{\mu} \frac{\partial P}{\partial z}(y^2 - h^2) + V_z \right] dy + \int_h^{h+H} \left[\frac{V_z \sinh M_z(h+H-y)}{\sinh(M_z H)} \right] dy + \int_h^{h+H}$$

$$\times \left[\frac{\varphi_2}{\mu} \frac{\partial P}{\partial z} \frac{1}{\sinh M_z H} (\sinh M_z(h+H-y) - \sinh M_z(h-y) - \sinh(M_z H)) \right] dy.$$

On integrating the above integrals and simplifying the expressions, we get the expression for the synovial fluid flux in pathological synovial joint in the z-direction.

$$Q_z = -\frac{\partial P}{\partial z} \left[\frac{1}{M_z^3 \mu'} \left(\tanh M_z H \left(M_z h - \tanh \frac{M_z H}{2} \right)^2 + M_z H + 2\tanh \frac{M_z H}{2} \right) + \frac{h^3}{3\mu} \right]. \quad (8)$$

The continuity equation for the hydrodynamic zone or fluid film region is

$$\frac{\partial u_1}{\partial x} + \frac{\partial v_1}{\partial z} + \frac{\partial w_1}{\partial y} = 0, \quad (9)$$

where w_1 is the velocity of synovial fluid in the fluid film along the y-direction.

The above continuity equation in integrated form is written as follows:

$$\frac{\partial Q_x}{\partial x} + \frac{\partial Q_z}{\partial z} + \frac{\partial w_1}{\partial y} = 0. \quad (10)$$

Integrating the above equation across the fluid film and using the boundary condition $w_1 = 0$ at $y = 0$ and $w_1 = V_s$ at $y = h$.

From Eqs. (7) and (8), the expression for the volumetric flux of synovial fluid in both directions is as follows:

$$Q_x = -\frac{\partial P}{\partial x} \left[\frac{1}{M_x^3 \mu'} \left(\tanh M_x H \left(M_x h - \tanh \frac{M_x H}{2} \right)^2 + M_x H + 2\tanh \frac{M_x H}{2} \right) + \frac{h^3}{3\mu} \right],$$

$$(11)$$

$$Q_z = -\frac{\partial P}{\partial z} \left[\frac{1}{M_z^3 \mu'} \left(\tanh M_z H \left(M_z h - \tanh \frac{M_z H}{2} \right)^2 + M_z H + 2\tanh \frac{M_z H}{2} \right) + \frac{h^3}{3\mu} \right].$$

$$(12)$$

Now putting the values of Q_x and Q_z in Eq. (10) which are given in Eqs. (11) and (12), we obtained the following expression:

$$\frac{\partial}{\partial x}\left[-\left\{\frac{1}{M_x^3\mu'}\left(\tanh M_xH\left(M_xh-\tanh\frac{M_xH}{2}\right)^2+M_xH+2\tanh\frac{M_xH}{2}\right)+\frac{h^3}{3\mu}\right\}\frac{\partial P}{\partial x}\right]$$

$$+\frac{\partial}{\partial z}\left[-\left\{\frac{1}{M_z^3\mu'}\left(\tanh M_zH\left(M_zh-\tanh\frac{M_zH}{2}\right)^2+M_zH+2\tanh\frac{M_zH}{2}\right)+\frac{h^3}{3\mu}\right\}\frac{\partial P}{\partial z}\right]$$

$$=-V_s. \tag{13}$$

This equation is the modified form of the Reynolds equation for squeezing film between articular cartilages approximated as parallel plates to obtain the fluid film's pressure and other important characteristics. We have considered the flow of synovial fluid in such a way that there is no change in pressure in the z-direction, and hence the rate of change of pressure in this direction will be zero. Therefore, we have $\frac{\partial p}{\partial z}=0$, and Eq. (13) reduces to the following equation:

$$\frac{\partial}{\partial x}\left[-\left\{\frac{1}{M_x^3\mu'}\left(\tanh M_xH\left(M_xh-\tanh\frac{M_xH}{2}\right)^2+M_xH+2\tanh\frac{M_xH}{2}\right)+\frac{h^3}{3\mu}\right\}\frac{\partial P}{\partial x}\right]$$

$$=-V_s. \tag{14}$$

The boundary conditions for the pressure in the x-direction are given by

$$\frac{\partial P}{\partial x}=0 \quad \text{at } x=0 \quad \text{and} \quad P=0 \quad \text{at } x=L_x. \tag{15}$$

Now we solve Eq. (14) using simple integration approach, and by applying the boundary conditions given in Eq. (15), we get the expression for the pressure in fluid film and articular cartilage, and the expression for pressure is as follows:

$$P(x)=\frac{V_s(L_x^2-x^2)}{2\left[\frac{1}{M_x^3\mu'}\left(\tanh M_xH\left(M_xh-\tanh\frac{M_xH}{2}\right)^2+M_xH+2\tanh\frac{M_xH}{2}\right)+\frac{h^3}{3\mu}\right]}. \tag{16}$$

The load capacity of the squeeze film is obtained by integrating pressure along the length of the porous medium. Therefore, we integrate the expression of pressure with respect to x across the length of the articular cartilage to obtain the expression for the load capacity in squeeze film formed in between the articular cartilages. Therefore, we have

$$W_x=\int_0^{L_x}P(x)dx. \tag{17}$$

By substituting the value of $P(x)$ from Eq. (16) into Eq. (17), we get the expression for the load capacity in squeeze film in between both articular cartilages and the expression for load capacity is given by

$$W_x = \int_0^{L_x} \frac{V_s(L_x^2 - x^2)}{2\left[\frac{1}{M_x^3\mu'}\left(\tanh M_x H\left(M_x h - \tanh\frac{M_x H}{2}\right)^2 + M_x H + 2\tanh\frac{M_x H}{2}\right) + \frac{h^3}{3\mu}\right]} dx.$$

On integrating the above expression and further simplifying it, we get the final expression for the load capacity of the squeeze film of the synovial joint. The load-carrying capacity is given as follows:

$$W_x = \frac{V_s L_x^3}{3\left[\frac{1}{M_x^3\mu'}\left(\tanh M_x H\left(M_x h - \tanh\frac{M_x H}{2}\right)^2 + M_x H + 2\tanh\frac{M_x H}{2}\right) + \frac{h^3}{3\mu}\right]}. \tag{18}$$

Squeeze velocity is the rate of change of fluid film thickness with respect to time and is given by $V_s = -(\frac{dh}{dt})$. By using the expression for squeeze velocity in Eq. (18) and integrating from the initial film thickness h_1 to the final film thickness h_2, we get the expression for squeeze time

$$T_x = \int_{h_1}^{h_2} \frac{L_x^3}{3W_x\left[\frac{1}{M_x^3\mu'}\left(\tanh M_x H\left(M_x h - \tanh\frac{M_x H}{2}\right)^2 + M_x H + 2\tanh\frac{M_x H}{2}\right) + \frac{h^3}{3\mu}\right]} dh.$$

$$\tag{19}$$

Here h_1 and h_2 denote the initial and final fluid film thickness formed in the synovial cavity.

To obtain the dimensionless expression for pressure, load capacity, and squeeze time, we shall use the following dimensionless variables:

$$\bar{x} = \frac{x}{L}, \quad \bar{L}_x = \frac{L_x}{L}, \quad \bar{h} = \frac{h}{h_0}, \quad \bar{h}_2 = \frac{h_2}{h_0}, \quad \bar{h}_1 = \frac{h_1}{h_0}, \quad \bar{H} = \frac{H}{h_0}, \quad \bar{\mu}' = \frac{\mu'}{\mu_0},$$

$$\bar{V}_s = \frac{V_s}{U}, \quad \bar{\mu} = \frac{\mu}{\mu_0}, \quad \bar{M}_x = \frac{M_x}{h_0}, \quad \bar{\varphi}_1 = \frac{\varphi_1}{h_0^2}, \quad \bar{W}_x = \frac{W_x}{\left(\frac{L^3}{\mu_0}\right)}, \quad \bar{T}_x = \frac{T_x}{\left(\frac{\mu_0 L}{W_x}\right)}, \tag{20}$$

where L, U, h_0 and μ_0 are the scaling parameters. The symbol L denotes the maximum possible length of the articular cartilage, U denotes the maximum squeezing velocity, h_0 denotes the maximum fluid film thickness and μ_0 denotes the maximum viscosity of the synovial fluid. The symbols with overbar signs represent the dimensionless expression for their respective notations.

We have used the above dimensionless scheme given in Eq. (20) to non-dimensionalize the expression of pressure, load capacity, and squeeze time given in Eqs. (16), (18), and (19) and obtained the expression for dimensionless pressure, dimensionless load capacity and dimensionless squeeze time.

The expressions for dimensionless pressure, dimensionless load capacity, and dimensionless squeeze time are given as follows:

$$\overline{P}(x) = \frac{\overline{V}_s U(\overline{L}_x^2 - \overline{x}^2)(\overline{M}_x^3 \overline{\mu}' \mu_0 h_0{}^4)}{2L\left[\tanh \overline{M}_x \overline{H} h_0^2 \left(\overline{M}_x \overline{H} h_0^2 - \tanh \frac{\overline{M}_x \overline{H} h_0^2}{2}\right)^2 + \overline{M}_x \overline{H} h_0^2 + 2\tanh \frac{\overline{M}_x \overline{H} h_0^2}{2}\right] + \frac{\overline{h}^3}{3\overline{\mu}\mu_0}},$$

$$\overline{W}_x = \frac{\overline{V}_s U \mu_0 \overline{L}_x^3}{3\left[\tanh \overline{M}_x \overline{H} h_0^2 \left(\overline{M}_x \overline{H} h_0^2 - \tanh \frac{\overline{M}_x \overline{H} h_0^2}{2}\right)^2 + \overline{M}_x \overline{H} h_0^2 + 2\tanh \frac{\overline{M}_x \overline{H} h_0^2}{2}\right] + \frac{\overline{h}^3}{3\overline{\mu}\mu_0}},$$

$$\overline{T}_x = \int_{h_0 \overline{h}_1}^{h_0 \overline{h}_2} \frac{1}{3\left[\tanh \overline{M}_x \overline{H} h_0^2 \left(\overline{M}_x \overline{H} h_0^2 - \tanh \frac{\overline{M}_x \overline{H} h_0^2}{2}\right)^2 + \overline{M}_x \overline{H} h_0^2 + 2\tanh \frac{\overline{M}_x \overline{H} h_0^2}{2}\right] + \frac{\overline{h}^3}{3\overline{\mu}\mu_0}} d\overline{h},$$

where $\overline{M}_x$ is the dimensionless form of the expression M_x, which is given by

$$\overline{M}_x = \frac{1}{h_0}\left(\frac{1}{\overline{\mu}' \overline{\varphi}_1}\right)^{1/2}.$$

The expressions mentioned above represent dimensionless properties of the squeeze film found in the synovial cavity of a diseased human knee joint. These properties, namely pressure, load-carrying capacity, and squeezing time, are critical in describing the behavior of squeeze films. To investigate the impact of various physiological parameters on these properties and how they change with these parameters, we have plotted the variations of pressure, load-carrying capacity, and squeezing time against these parameters.

Results and Discussion

This study presents the characteristics of squeeze film formed in between the articular cartilages of the diseased human knee joints. In order to study the characteristics of the squeeze film, modified form of the well-known Reynolds equation for squeeze films has been obtained and subsequently derived the expression for pressure, load carrying capacity, and squeeze time. Further, dimensionless expressions for pressure, load capacity, and squeeze time have been obtained. The squeeze time is the time taken to reduce the film thickness from an initial value to a particular value. In this present case, we have considered the squeeze time as the time to reduce the film thickness to zero so that the articular cartilages rub with each other. The effects of various parameters on pressure distribution in squeeze film, load capacity, and squeeze time for axial directions have been studied. The effects of permeability, viscosity, squeeze velocity, and fluid film thickness on pressure variation are considered. Meanwhile, the effects of permeability, squeeze velocity, and viscosity on the load capacity of squeeze film also have been obtained. On the other hand, the only parameter affecting the squeeze time is the viscosity studied in this work. The variation of dimensionless pressure with dimensionless axial distance for different values of fluid film thickness, the viscosity of the synovial fluid, the permeability of articular cartilage, and squeeze velocity has been shown. Further, the variation of dimensionless load capacity with dimensionless fluid film thickness for different values of permeability of articular cartilage and viscosity of synovial fluid has been plotted. Lastly, the variation of dimensionless squeeze time with dimensionless articular cartilage length and thickness for different values of the viscosity of synovial fluid has been shown.

Figures 4–7 show the variation of dimensionless pressure $\overline{P}(x)$ with dimensionless axial distance $\overline{x}$ for these parameters, whereas Figs. 8–10 show the variation of dimensionless load capacity $\overline{W}_x$ with dimensionless fluid film thickness $\overline{h}$, for different values of permeability, viscosity and squeeze velocity. Figures 11 and 12 show the variation of dimensionless squeeze time $\overline{T}_x$ with dimensionless cartilage thickness $\overline{H}$ and dimensionless cartilage length $\overline{L}_x$. The value of dimensionless pressure $\overline{P}(x)$ decreases with axial distance $\overline{x}$ for all the parameters. The pressure $\overline{P}(x)$ in fluid film decreases when the value of dimensionless permeability

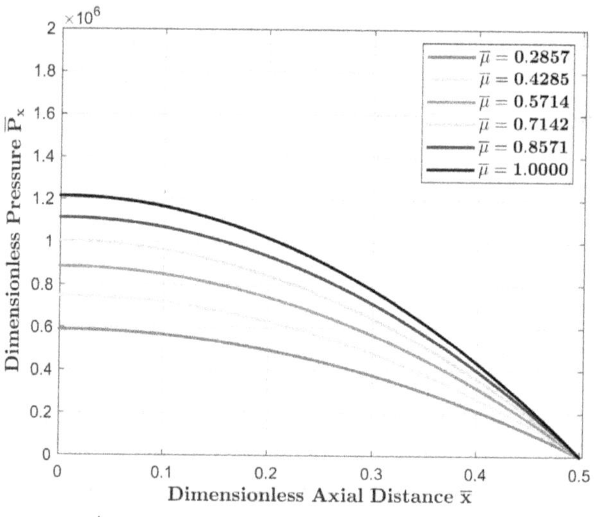

Fig. 4.   Pressure variation with axial distance for different values of viscosity.

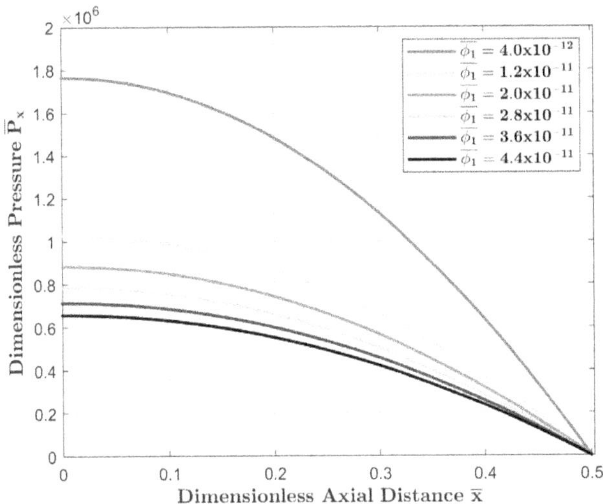

Fig. 5.   Pressure variation with axial distance for different values of cartilage permeability.

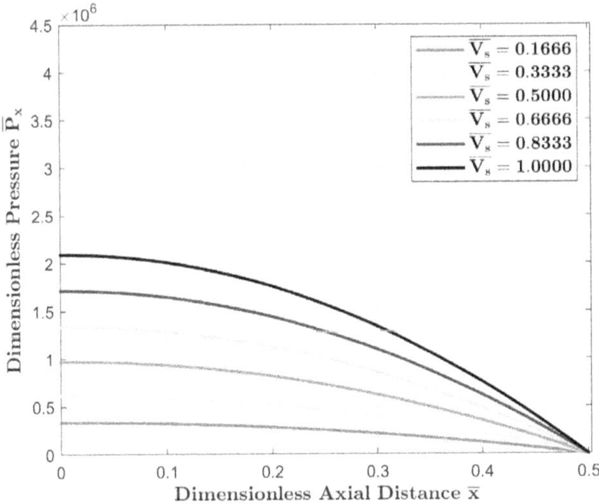

Fig. 6.   Pressure variation with axial distance for different values of squeeze velocity.

$\overline{\varphi}_1$ and dimensionless fluid film thickness $\overline{h}$ increases and it increases when the value of dimensionless squeeze velocity $\overline{V}_s$ and the viscosity μ of synovial fluid increases. These results are similar with the results given in Kudenatti *et al.* (2013). The value of dimensionless load capacity $\overline{W}_x$ decreases with an increase in

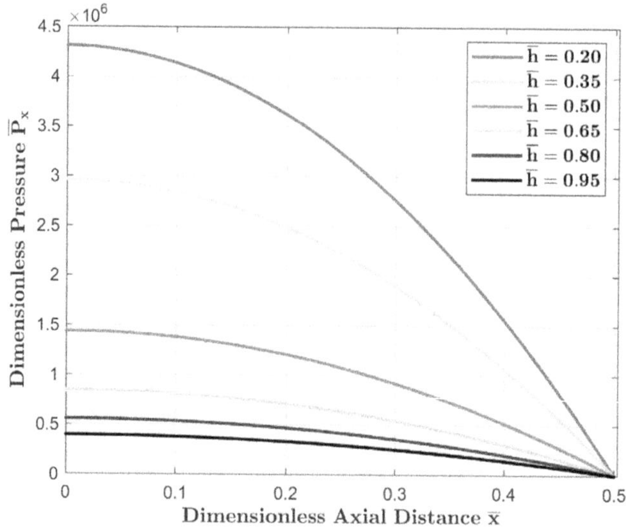

Fig. 7.   Pressure variation with axial distance for different values of fluid film thickness.

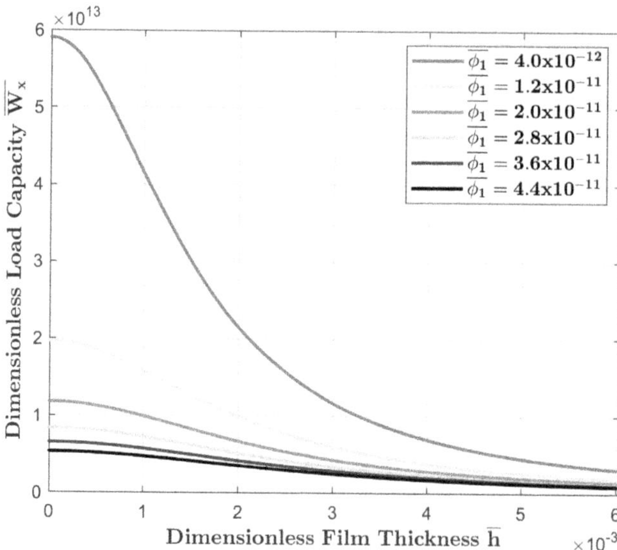

Fig. 8.   Load capacity variation with film thickness for different values of cartilage permeability.

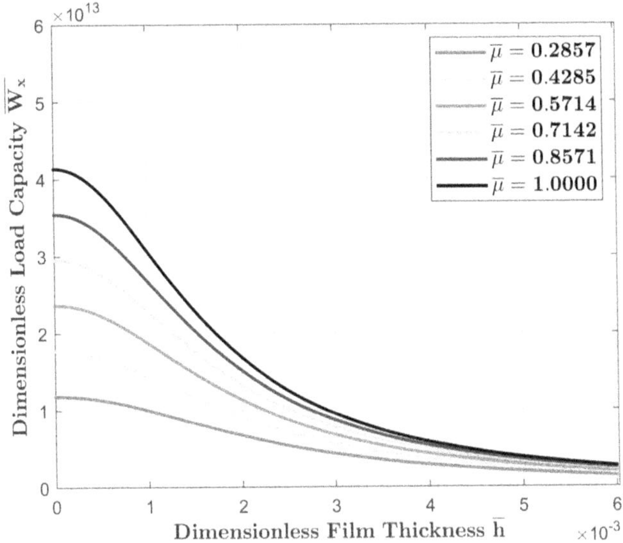

Fig. 9. Load capacity variation with film thickness for different values of viscosity.

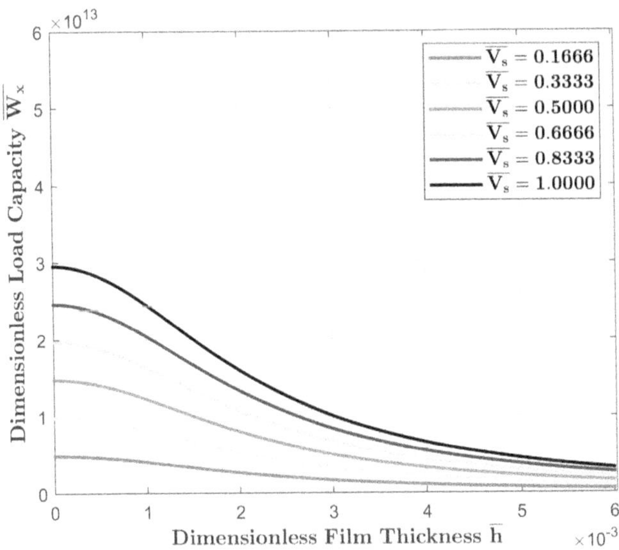

Fig. 10. Load capacity variation with film thickness for different values of squeeze velocity.

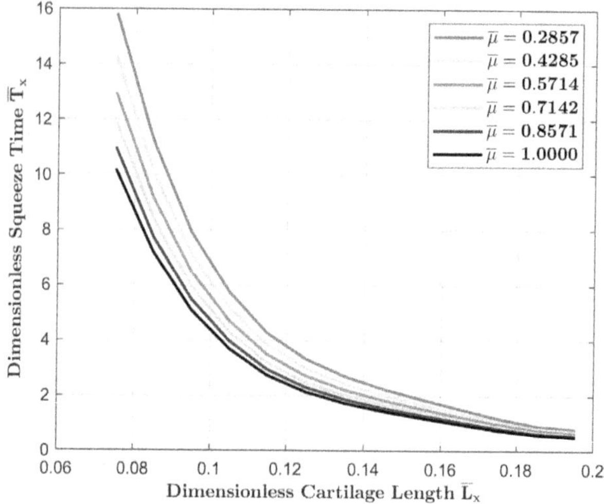

Fig. 11.   Squeeze time variation with cartilage length for different values of viscosity.

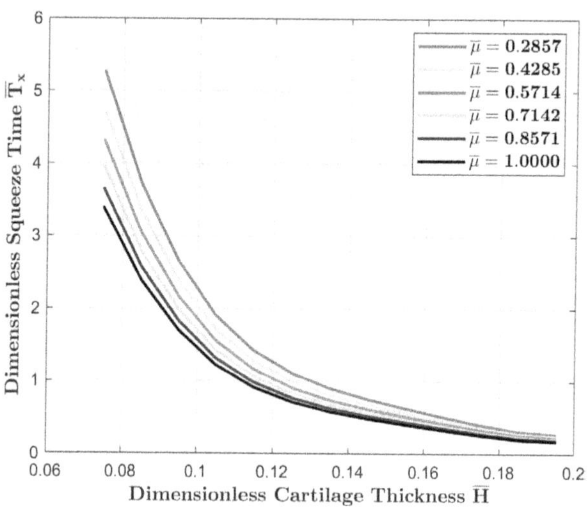

Fig. 12.   Squeeze time variation with cartilage thickness for different values of viscosity.

dimensionless fluid film thickness $\bar{h}$ generally, whereas the value of dimensionless load capacity $\overline{W}_x$ increases as the value of viscosity μ and dimensionless squeeze velocity $\overline{V}_s$ increases and this dimensionless load capacity $\overline{W}_x$ increases when the permeability $\bar{\varphi}_1$ of articular cartilage decreases. Our results for load capacity are similar with Naduvinamani and Savitramma (2013) and Kumar and Raghavendra (2015). Figures 11 and 12 show the variation of dimensionless squeeze time $\overline{T}_x$ with dimensionless cartilage length $\overline{L}_x$ and cartilage thickness $\overline{H}$ for different values of viscosity of the synovial fluid. Squeeze time $\overline{T}_x$ decreases with cartilage length $\overline{L}_x$ as well as cartilage thickness $\overline{H}$. The value of squeeze time $\overline{T}_x$ decreases as the value of viscosity of synovial fluid increases for both the cases. The results we obtained for squeeze time are similar to those obtained by Sinha *et al.* (1983). Squeeze time decreases when the value of the thickness of the articular cartilage and the length of the articular cartilage increases. Based on the results obtained in this work, it might be easy to get a good insight into the condition of the diseased human knee joint. The diseased human knee joint goes through various biochemical and biomechanical changes. Due to these conditions, the permeability of articular cartilage increases while the viscosity of synovial fluid decreases (Hays, 1963).

The pressure in the knee joint is more during exercise and diseased conditions in comparison to resting and normal conditions. Due to this increased pressure, hypoxic reperfusion free radicals are generated in the knee joint resulting in the damage of articular cartilage tissue. Therefore, increased pressure in the synovial joint is a marker of chronic joint disease. We already observed that pressure increases when squeezing velocity and viscosity increase, which clearly shows that during movement and disease, pressure increases. On the other hand, pressure decreases when film thickness and permeability increase, which also verifies the diseased and mobility condition. Therefore, we can conclude that the mobility of the human knee joint decreases in the diseased condition due to increased pressure. It can also be concluded that the ability of the human knee joint to bear loads decreases in diseased conditions and increases during movement, as the permeability is more and viscosity is less in disease conditions while the squeeze velocity is more during movement. Squeeze time increases in diseased joints as it decreases with the thickness of articular cartilage and the viscosity of the synovial fluid, and these values decrease in the diseased condition of the human knee joint (Naduvinamani *et al.*, 2004).

The squeeze film properties of synovial joints can provide important information for the diagnosis of synovial joint diseases. Synovial fluid is a key component of these properties and plays a crucial role in joint lubrication and nutrition. Changes in the properties of synovial fluid can indicate the presence of synovial joint disease and help clinicians in the diagnosis of the conditions. In patients with osteoarthritis, the thickness and composition of synovial fluid change due to the degeneration of articular cartilage and other joint tissues. The altered properties of synovial fluid can reduce its ability to lubricate the joint and may increase friction and wear, leading to joint pain, stiffness, and reduced mobility. Measuring the thickness and composition of synovial fluid can provide an indication of the severity of the disease and help guide treatment decisions. In patients with rheumatoid arthritis, the properties of synovial fluid are also altered due to the inflammatory response. The fluid becomes thinner and contains higher levels of inflammatory markers, which can help in the diagnosis of the disease. In joint injury or surgery cases, synovial fluid may be reduced, leading to increased friction and wear in the joint. By understanding the lubricating properties of the fluid, clinicians can develop treatments to enhance the properties of synovial fluid and improve joint function. Overall, the squeeze film properties of synovial joints can be useful in the diagnosis of synovial joint diseases. By analyzing the properties of synovial fluid, clinicians can detect early signs of joint disease, monitor disease progression, and make informed treatment decisions.

The current model is not definitive and can be improved by introducing new assumptions and hypotheses. Due to the computational challenges involved, we have restricted our analysis of the modified Reynolds equation to a one-dimensional context. The characteristics of articular cartilages and synovial fluid differ depending on various factors, which means that the friction coefficient of synovial joints measured *in vivo* cannot be identified through *in vitro* testing. This makes it difficult to develop synovial joint models with precise specifications. The actual geometry of synovial joints is not identical to parallel plates; therefore, cylindrical surfaces may be a better approximation for articular cartilage. Future studies will need to consider the interaction between cylindrical geometry and synovial fluid as a biological lubricant to assess pressure distribution, load capacity of squeeze film, and squeezing time of the articular cartilage.

3. Conclusion

In this study, the modified Reynolds equation for the flow of the synovial fluid in diseased human knee joints has been studied. We have theoretically analyzed the formation of a squeeze film between the articular cartilages and studied the flow of synovial fluid. We have modeled the articular cartilages as parallel plates and studied the impact of various parameters, such as viscosity, permeability, and thickness of the fluid film, on the characteristics of the squeeze film. We have concluded that these parameters significantly affect the properties of the fluid film, including pressure and load capacity. Further, we have studied the effect of squeeze velocity, fluid film thickness, articular cartilage permeability, and synovial fluid viscosity on pressure and load capacity. It has been observed that the pressure in the squeeze film increases with an increase in the viscosity of the synovial fluid and the squeeze velocity of the articular cartilage. At the same time, the pressure decreases when the permeability of the articular cartilages and the thickness of the fluid film in between the articular cartilages increase. The load-carrying capacity (the ability to sustain/bear load) increases with the viscosity of the synovial fluid and decreases with the increase of permeability of articular cartilages. It has been observed by the profile shown in the figures that the load capacity decreases as the dimensionless fluid film thickness increases. Also, by observing the same figures, it can be seen that the load capacity increases with an increase in viscosity and dimensionless squeeze velocity. However, the load capacity decreases when the value of dimensionless permeability increases. It is also observed that the squeeze time does depend on the viscosity of the synovial fluid and the length and thickness of the articular cartilages of the knee joint. Squeeze time decreases when the value of the thickness of the articular cartilage and the length of the articular cartilage increases.

Based on the results obtained in this study, we can conclude that the condition of a diseased human knee joint can be better understood by analyzing the biochemical and biomechanical changes that occur, such as increased permeability of articular cartilages and decreased viscosity of the synovial fluid. Increased pressure in the joint during exercise and disease can lead to the generation of free radicals and damage to the articular cartilage tissue. The study also found that pressure increases with increased squeeze velocity and viscosity, but decreases with increased film thickness and permeability, indicating decreased mobility and load-bearing ability in diseased conditions. Squeeze time was also found to increase in diseased joints due to changes in the thickness of articular cartilage and viscosity of the synovial fluid.

References

Bazrov, BM (2010) Classification of joints, *Russ. Eng. Res.* **30**, 399–403.
Coffman, J (1980) Synovial fluid, *Vet. Med. Small Anim. Clin.* **75**, 1403–1406.
Damiano, J and Bardin, T (2004) Synovial fluid, EMC-Rhumatol.-Orthoped. **1**, 2–16.
Davies, DV (1966) Properties of synovial fluid, *Proc. Inst. Mech. Eng.* **8**, 25–29.
Deheri, G, Patel, H and Patel, R (2011) Load carrying capacity and time height relation for squeeze film between rough porous rectangular plates, *Ann. Fac. Eng. Hunedoara* **9**, 33.
Dintenfass, L (1963) Lubrication in synovial joints, *Nature* **197**, 496–497.
Gibbs, DA, Merrill, EW, Smith, KA and Balazs, EA (1968) Rheology of hyaluronic acid, *Biopolymers* **6**, 777–791.
Hays, DF (1963). Squeeze films for rectangular plates, *J. Fluids Eng. Trans. ASME* **85**, 243–246.
Hui, AY, McCarty, WJ, Masuda, K, Firestein, GS and Sah, RL (2012) A systems biology approach to synovial joint lubrication in health, injury, and disease. *Wiley Interdiscip. Rev. Syst. Biol. Med.* **4**(1), 15–37, https://doi.org/10.1002/wsbm.157.

Klein, J (2006) Molecular mechanisms of synovial joint lubrication, *Proc. Inst. Mech. Eng. Part J: J. Eng. Tribol.* **220**(8), 691–710, doi:10.1243/13506501JET143.

Kudenatti, RB, Murulidhara, N and Patil, HP (2013) Numerical study of squeeze film lubrication between porous and rough rectangular plates, *J. Porous Media* **16**, 183–192.

Kumar, JV and Raghavendra, R (2015) Effects of surface roughness in squeeze film lubrication of spherical bearings, *Proc. Eng.* **127**, 955–962.

Mathieu, P, Conrozier, T, Vignon, E, Rozand, Y, Rinaudo, M (2009) Rheologic behavior of osteoarthritic synovial fluid after addition of hyaluronic acid: A pilot study, *Clinical Orthopaedics and Related Research* **467**(11), 3002–3009, doi: 10.1007/s11999-009-0867-x.

Naduvinamani, NB, Fathima, ST and PS Hiremath (2004) On the squeeze effect of lubricants with additives between rough porous rectangular plates, *ZAMM Z. Angew. Math. Mech.* **84**, 825–834.

Naduvinamani, NB and Savitramma, GK (2013) Squeeze film lubrication between rough poroelastic rectangular plates with micropolar fluid: A special reference to the study of synovial joint lubrication, *ISRN Tribol.* 1–9.

Ogston, AG and Stanier, JE (1953) The physiological function of hyaluronic acid in synovial fluid; viscous, elastic and lubricant properties, *J. Physiol.* **119**, 244–252.

Ruggiero, A (2020) Milestones in natural lubrication of synovial joints, *Front. Mech. Eng.* **6**, 52, doi:10.3389/fmech.2020.00052.

Sadique, M, Shah, S, Sharma, S and Islam, S (2023) Effect of significant parameters on squeeze film characteristics in pathological synovial joints, *Mathematics* **11**(6), 1468, https://doi.org/10.3390/math11061468.

Shukla, JB (1978) A new theory of lubrication for rough surfaces, *Wear* **49**, 33–42.

Singh, SP, Chadda, GC and Sinha, AK (1988) A model for micropolar fluid film mechanism with reference to human joints, *Indian J. Pure Appl. Math.* **19**, 384–394.

Sinha, P, Singh, C and Prasad, KR (1982) Lubrication of human joints — a microcontinuum approach, *Wear* **80**, 159–181.

Sinha, P, Singh, C and Prasad, KR (1983) Viscosity variation considering cavitation in a journal bearing lubricant containing additives, *Wear* **86**, 43–56.

Verschoor, H (1951) Experimental data on the viscous force exerted by a flowing fluid on a dense swarm of particles, *Appl. Sci. Res.* **2**, 155–161.

Wu, H (1972) An analysis of the squeeze film between porous rectangular plates, *J. Tribol.* **94**, 64–68.

CHAPTER 5

A Scoping Review of Current Methods and Limitations for Modeling and Evaluating Ligamentous Structures[a]

Christine D. Walck[*,‡], Braden C. Fleming[†], Aspen E. Taylor[*],
Pablo Vilches Mangada[*] and Anthony T. Dioguardi[*]

*Department of Mechanical Engineering,
College of Engineering, Embry-Riddle Aeronautical University,
Daytona Beach, FL 32114, USA

†School of Engineering, Brown University,
Providence, RI 02912, USA
‡christine.walck@erau.edu

Recently, scientists have utilized a range of techniques in the attempt to model ligamentous structures, which play a vital role in the functioning of the human body. Therefore, our objective is to conduct a systematic scoping review that evaluates the scope of 163 journals pertaining to computational modeling of ligaments, while also assessing the limitations associated with each method. These limitations encompass various aspects, including anatomical considerations, subject specificity, viscoelasticity, mechanical properties, model-specific factors, and limitations related to medical imaging. The guiding question for this review is: What are the existing limitations in the surveyed literature regarding ligament modeling and methods, specifically with regard to time variance and environmental hazards? A search of PubMed/MEDLINE, Web of Science (WoS), and ScienceDirect was conducted following the scoping review methodology recommended by the Joanna Briggs Institute (JBI) for evidence-based healthcare. After applying the inclusion and exclusion criteria, 74 full-text articles were analyzed, revealing that each method possesses its own set of limitations and may not comprehensively encompass all aspects of ligament properties. Nevertheless, despite these limitations, the majority of these methods exhibit the ability to produce reliable outcomes.

Keywords: Computed tomography; ligament model; magnetic resonance imaging; musculoskeletal models; computational models; mathematical models; finite element models; constitutive models; mechanistic modeling.

---

‡Corresponding author.
[a]This article was previously published in *World Scientific Annual Review of Biomechanics*. Vol: 1, (2023) 2330005 (56 pages).

1. Introduction

Ligaments are an important biological aspect of the human body. They are fibrous connective tissues that connect bones and provide stability to joints. Ligaments consist primarily of collagen fibers, which give them strength and flexibility (Frank, 2004). Ligaments play a crucial role in providing stability and guiding the movement of diarthrodial joints, such as the knee, hip, and shoulder, which are known for their high mobility. Their primary function is to restrict excessive movement and maintain the joint within its normal range of motion when external forces are applied. This important function helps prevent joint dislocation or damage, ensuring optimal joint function and overall joint health (Frank, 2004; Jung *et al.*, 2009; Walck, 2019; Peel *et al.*, 2023). Additionally, ligaments act as mechanoreceptors, providing sensory information about joint position and movement. They contain specialized nerve endings called mechanoreceptors, which detect mechanical stimuli and contribute to proprioception. Proprioception is the body's ability to sense its position, orientation, and movement in space. Ligaments play a significant role in providing feedback to the central nervous system about joint position and motion, aiding in coordination, balance, and posture (Dhillon *et al.*, 2012).

Ligaments exhibit viscoelastic behavior, which means they demonstrate both viscous and elastic responses to applied forces. The viscoelastic properties of ligaments are depicted in Fig. 1. The viscous component refers to the time-dependent deformation and energy dissipation, while the elastic component represents the ability of the ligament to return to its original shape after deformation. This combination of viscosity and elasticity allows ligaments to absorb and distribute forces, providing stability and preventing joint damage (Solomonow, 2009). Furthermore, every time a viscoelastic material is under load there is an energy loss, known as hysteresis (Farrell, 1999; Adeeb *et al.*, 2004). These types of materials also have

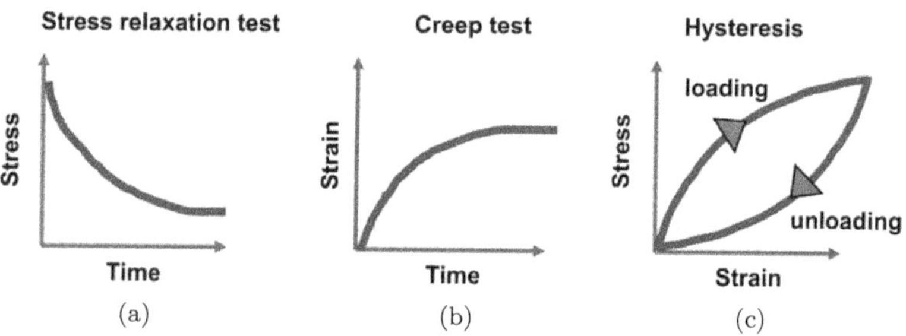

Fig. 1.   Characteristics of a viscoelastic material include: (a) creep, (b) stress relaxation, and (c) hysteresis.
Source: Mierke (2021).

history-dependent mechanics resulting in different load–strain curves depending on the loading rate (Zhang *et al.*, 2016). This time-dependent behavior of materials is crucial in determining their stiffness. When a constant change in length is applied to a material and maintained over time, a decrease in force, known as load relaxation, is observed (Screen, 2008). Conversely, when a constant force is applied to a material for a period of time, an increase in length occurs, which is referred to as creep (Zhou *et al.*, 2021). These phenomena, load relaxation and creep, demonstrate the material's time-dependent response and are significant factors in understanding the mechanical properties of the material.

Ligaments exhibit a hierarchical structure composed of collagen fibers arranged in a crimp pattern. When subjected to loading, the crimp pattern of the ligament straightens out, resulting in the initial toe region of the stress–strain curve. As the fibers further elongate, the ligament enters the linear region of the curve. At the end of this linear region, microscopic failures start to occur within the ligament structure. These failures can progress and ultimately lead to macroscopic failures or ruptures if additional loading is applied. This stress–strain behavior highlights the progressive response of ligaments under increasing loads and the potential for failure if the mechanical limits of the ligament are exceeded (Adeeb *et al.*, 2004; Zhang *et al.*, 2016).

Understanding the viscoelastic behavior of ligaments is crucial for accurately modeling their mechanical properties and predicting their response to different loading conditions. Incorporating these viscoelastic properties into computational models can improve the accuracy of simulations and help researchers gain a deeper understanding of ligament function, injury mechanisms, and rehabilitation strategies (Peters *et al.*, 2018). As a result, an initial search was performed on PubMed/MEDLINE, Web of Science (WoS), and ScienceDirect databases. Despite conducting an extensive search, no recent systematic reviews, ongoing studies, or scoping reviews that specifically address the topic were found beyond the year 2007 (Weiss and Gardiner, 2011). However, significant progress has been made in computational modeling techniques for ligaments since then. These advancements encompass various approaches, such as medical imaging methods (Blemker *et al.*, 2007), mechanistic (Kazemi *et al.*, 2013), musculoskeletal (Blemker *et al.*, 2007; Marra *et al.*, 2015), finite element (FE) (Kim *et al.*, 2018), continuum (Tian *et al.*, 2010), and mathematical modeling (Di Gregorio *et al.*, 2007). These developments signify the evolving landscape of ligament modeling and the diverse range of methodologies being employed in this field. The objective of this scoping review is to assess the extent of the literature associated with the computational modeling of ligaments, and the limitations that are involved with these methods.

The research question that guided this review is: What limitations exist in the surveyed literature concerning ligament modeling and methods, particularly considering the aspects of time variance and environmental hazards?

2. Methods

The proposed scoping review has been conducted in accordance with the Joanna Briggs Institute (JBI) methodology for scoping reviews (Aromataris *et al.*, 2015), defining the inclusion criteria as considering peer-reviewed journal articles with a population of medical professionals performing any type of analysis or modeling of ligamentous structures within the context of computational model modeling. The studies are grouped by experimental, quasi-experimental, analytical, descriptive, and qualitative studies.

2.1. *Search strategy and information sources*

The search strategy employed in this review aims to identify both published and unpublished studies. A three-step approach is implemented to ensure comprehensive coverage. Initially, a preliminary search is conducted on PubMed/MEDLINE, WoS, and ScienceDirect databases using specific keywords and index terms related to the topic. This initial search helps identify relevant articles based on the information contained in their titles and abstracts. Subsequently, a comprehensive search strategy is developed, incorporating the identified keywords and index terms, for each relevant database or information source. The search strategy details can be found in Appendix A. Furthermore, the reference lists of all included studies are carefully examined to identify any additional relevant sources of evidence that may have been missed during the initial search process. This multi-step search strategy is designed to maximize the retrieval of relevant studies and ensure the inclusion of a wide range of literature sources in the review.

2.2. *Data selection process*

After completing the search, all identified citations were compiled and uploaded into JBI Software. Duplicate citations were then removed to ensure a clean dataset. Subsequently, two independent reviewers conducted a thorough screening of the titles and abstracts of the identified citations. This screening process aimed to assess the relevance of each citation against the predetermined inclusion criteria for the review. By involving two reviewers, the screening process becomes more robust and minimizes potential bias, leading to a more objective evaluation of the sources. This rigorous approach enhances the reliability and validity of the review's findings.

Following the title and abstract screening, the relevant sources were obtained in their entirety, and their citation details were imported into JBI SUMARI, which is a software tool developed by JBI in Adelaide, Australia. JBI SUMARI is specifically designed to support systematic reviews and evidence synthesis. It serves as a comprehensive platform for researchers to manage the review process, evaluate the quality of studies, and analyze and synthesize the gathered information. By utilizing JBI SUMARI, researchers can streamline the review workflow and maintain a well-organized database of included studies. The software facilitates the analysis and synthesis of data, enabling researchers to extract meaningful insights and draw robust conclusions. JBI SUMARI's systematic and structured approach to evidence synthesis promotes transparency and rigor, ensuring a high-quality and reliable review process. It serves as a valuable tool in the systematic review journey, enhancing efficiency and facilitating evidence-based decision-making (Aromataris *et al.*, 2015).

The subsequent stage of the review process involves a comprehensive assessment of the full text of the selected citations in accordance with the predetermined inclusion criteria. This evaluation is carried out by two independent reviewers, ensuring a meticulous examination of each source (inter-rater reliability: $K = 0.98$). In the event of any discrepancies or disagreements between the reviewers, they are resolved through thorough discussion or, if necessary, with the involvement of an additional reviewer to reach a consensus. During the assessment of the full-text articles, the reviewers carefully analyze the content to determine if they meet the specific criteria set for the scoping review. Sources that do not meet the inclusion criteria are excluded, and the reasons for their exclusion are diligently documented and reported in the scoping review. This transparency in the selection process enables readers to comprehend the rationale behind the inclusion or exclusion of each source.

Upon completion of the full-text assessment, a comprehensive report detailing the results of the search and the study inclusion process is presented in the final scoping review. The report adheres to the PRISMA 2020 (Preferred Reporting Items for Systematic Reviews and Meta-Analyses) guidelines, which provide a standardized framework for reporting systematic reviews. Following these guidelines ensures transparency, clarity, and consistency in presenting the review process and findings (Page *et al.*, 2021). The scoping review encompasses essential information such as the total number of identified citations, the number of citations included at each stage of screening, and the rationale behind the exclusion of citations during the full-text assessment. Additionally, the final scoping review presents a comprehensive and in-depth summary of the included studies, highlighting their key characteristics, and elucidating any pertinent findings or emerging themes derived from the synthesis of the evidence. By adhering to this rigorous and transparent process, the scoping review guarantees the selection of pertinent studies, fostering a comprehensive overview of the available evidence pertaining to the research topic. This approach ensures the inclusion of relevant and reliable information, enabling readers to gain a thorough understanding of the existing literature in the field.

2.3. *Data collection process*

During the data extraction phase of the scoping review, two independent reviewers meticulously extract pertinent details from the included papers. The extracted data encompasses various aspects, including information about the participants, concept, context, study methods, and key findings that directly address the review questions. Throughout the data extraction process, modifications and revisions are made as required to ensure the accurate representation of all relevant information.

In cases where disagreements arise between the reviewers during data extraction, a collaborative discussion is held to reach a consensus. If necessary, an additional reviewer may be involved to provide their perspective and help resolve any discrepancies. This rigorous approach promotes consistency, reduces the potential for bias, and ensures the reliability of the extracted data. In the case of seeking the limitations of existing ligament modeling methods, the reviewers specifically focused on identifying and documenting the factors that contribute to decreased accuracy or inconsistent results. The objective is to highlight the generalized, high-level limitations that characterize these modeling methods and lead to a loss in precision.

The identified limitations may include the factors mentioned earlier, such as inaccurate insertion sites of ligaments, neglecting viscoelasticity, overlooking the zero-load length parameter, modeling ligaments as straight lines, disregarding time-dependent effects, and the absence of intrinsic and extrinsic factors in the models. Other limitations specific to the reviewed studies may also be identified during the extraction process.

By systematically documenting and analyzing these limitations, the scoping review aims to provide a comprehensive understanding of the challenges and drawbacks associated with existing ligament modeling methods. This information can help guide future research and development in the field, with the goal of improving the accuracy and reliability of ligament modeling approaches.

3. Results

3.1. *Study selection*

In the study selection process, a total of 163 papers were identified through the search strategy. After conducting title and abstract screening, 70 studies were excluded because they either did not contain relevant information about the modeling of ligaments or were duplicate studies.

During the full-text screening, an additional 19 studies were excluded. The primary reason for their exclusion was the lack of discussion on the limitations of computational modeling of ligaments. It appears that these studies did not adequately address or provide insights into the challenges and drawbacks associated with ligament modeling methods. As a result of the selection process, a total of 74 studies were included in this systematic review. These studies were deemed relevant and suitable for providing insights into the limitations of computational modeling approaches for ligaments.

The inclusion of these 74 studies in the systematic review will enable a comprehensive examination of the existing literature and provide a valuable understanding of the limitations that characterize ligament modeling methods. By analyzing these limitations, the review can identify areas for improvement and guide future research in developing more accurate and reliable computational models of ligaments.

Figure 2 depicts the PRISMA workflow for this study.

3.2. *Characteristics of included studies*

The included studies are expected to discuss the development of computational ligament models and explore and represent their limitations. By doing so, these studies acknowledge and address the challenges associated with accurately representing the complex structures and properties of ligaments through computational modeling. The discussion of limitations in the included studies is crucial because it allows researchers to identify and highlight the factors that hinder the accurate representation of ligaments. These limitations may include the factors mentioned earlier, such as inaccurate insertion sites, neglecting viscoelasticity, overlooking the zero-load length parameter, modeling ligaments as straight lines, disregarding time-dependent effects, and the exclusion of intrinsic and extrinsic factors.

By recognizing and discussing these limitations, researchers contribute to the understanding of the current state of computational ligament modeling and the

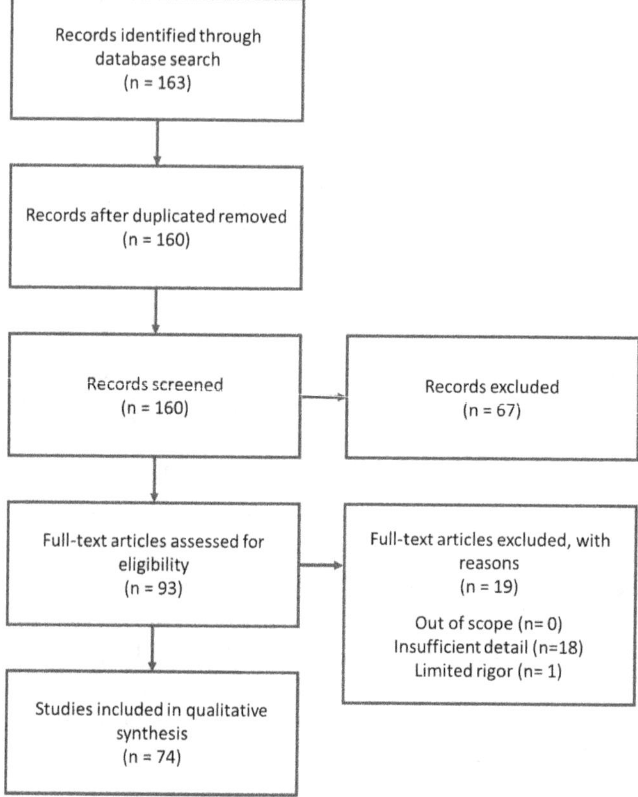

Fig. 2.   The PRISMA workflow for this study.

challenges that need to be addressed. It helps to identify areas where improvements and advancements are needed to enhance the accuracy and fidelity of ligament models. Through the systematic review, the collective findings from the included studies provide valuable insights into the limitations that exist in the current computational modeling of ligaments. This knowledge serves as a foundation for future research to develop more comprehensive and accurate models that better represent the complex nature of ligaments and their properties.

3.3. *Review findings*

3.3.1. *Anatomical limitations*

The anatomical limitations of computational models of ligaments are indeed significant factors that affect their accuracy. Several studies have pointed out specific limitations related to the representation of ligament anatomy in these models (Dhillon *et al.*, 2012; Marra *et al.*, 2015; Kim *et al.*, 2018; Di Gregorio *et al.*, 2007).

One common limitation is the representation of ligaments as straight lines between their origin and insertion points. This simplification fails to capture the true anatomy of ligaments, which attach over a finite area of bone and often wrap around the bones. This inaccurate representation can lead to simulation errors and a lack of fidelity in the model's behavior (Dhillon *et al.*, 2012; Marra *et al.*, 2015; Kim *et al.*, 2018). Additionally, some musculoskeletal models overlook the zero-load length parameter of ligaments. The zero-load length is an essential parameter that determines the initial tension or pre-stress in the ligament bundle. Neglecting this parameter can result in inaccurate representation of the ligament's behavior and compromise the accuracy of the model (Di Gregorio *et al.*, 2007). The anatomical limitations highlight the need for more sophisticated computational models that can better capture the complex and three-dimensional nature of ligaments. By incorporating more accurate anatomical representations, such as accounting for the finite area of attachment and wrapping around the bones, and considering the zero-load length parameter, the accuracy and realism of ligament models can be improved.

The anatomical limitations highlight the need for more sophisticated computational models that can better capture the complex and three-dimensional nature of ligaments. By incorporating more accurate anatomical representations, such as accounting for the finite area of attachment and wrapping around the bones, and considering the zero-load length parameter, the accuracy and realism of ligament models can be improved.

Future research should aim to address these anatomical limitations and develop computational models that more closely resemble the true anatomical characteristics of ligaments. By doing so, we can enhance our understanding of ligament function, injury mechanisms, and rehabilitation strategies, leading to advancements in the biomechanical field.

3.3.2. *Subject-specific data limitations*

Another limitation often observed in computational model studies of ligaments is the lack of inclusion of subject-specific experimental data. Obtaining and incorporating subject-specific data into computational models can be a time-consuming and resource-intensive process, which leads to its omission in many studies (Baldwin *et al.*, 2012). Subject-specific data refers to data collected from individual subjects, such as their anatomical measurements, tissue properties, and loading conditions. Including subject-specific data allows for a more personalized and accurate representation of the biomechanical behavior of ligaments within an individual (Carey *et al.*, 2014).

However, acquiring subject-specific data involves various challenges, including the need for imaging techniques, data processing, and validation (Lim *et al.*, 2022). It requires time and effort to collect and process the necessary data for each subject, which can be impractical in certain research contexts or for large-scale studies. As a result, many computational model studies resort to using generic or average data that may not accurately represent the specific characteristics of an individual's ligaments. This can limit the precision and individualized nature of the models, potentially affecting their accuracy and applicability to real-world scenarios (Willemink *et al.*, 2020).

Another limitation often observed in computational model studies of ligaments is the lack of inclusion of subject-specific experimental data. Obtaining and incorporating subject-specific data into computational models can be a time-consuming and resource-intensive process, which leads to its omission in many studies (Di Gregorio *et al.*, 2007). Subject-specific data refers to data collected from individual subjects, such as their anatomical measurements, tissue properties, and loading conditions. Including subject-specific data allows for a more personalized and accurate representation of the biomechanical behavior of ligaments within an individual.

However, acquiring subject-specific data involves various challenges, including the need for imaging techniques, data processing, and validation. It requires time and effort to collect and process the necessary data for each subject, which can be impractical in certain research contexts or for large-scale studies.

As a result, many computational model studies resort to using generic or average data that may not accurately represent the specific characteristics of an individual's ligaments. This can limit the precision and individualized nature of the models, potentially affecting their accuracy and applicability to real-world scenarios. Overcoming the limitations related to subject-specific data collection is an area of ongoing research. Efforts are being made to develop efficient techniques for obtaining subject-specific data, such as advanced imaging methods and data integration algorithms. By incorporating more subject-specific data into computational models, we can improve their accuracy and better tailor them to individual patients or study subjects. It is important for future research to address this limitation by striving to include subject-specific experimental data whenever possible, as it can significantly enhance the accuracy and reliability of computational models of ligaments.

3.3.3. *Viscoelasticity limitations*

During the development of computational models, it has been observed that the viscoelastic effects of ligaments are sometimes minimized or ignored in experiments (Yang *et al.*, 2010). This disregard for ligament viscoelasticity reduces the precision of the results obtained. In studies using finite element models, the consideration of ligament viscoelasticity and pre-straining properties has been neglected (Hamidrad *et al.*, 2021). However, in order to produce accurate results, it is important to properly characterize the visco-hyperelastic biomechanical behavior of ligaments in constitutive models (Jiang *et al.*, 2015). Unfortunately, ligament viscoelasticity is also commonly ignored in musculoskeletal models (Shelburne and Pandy, 1997) and mechanistic modeling (Barrett and Callaghan, 2017). This omission hampers the accurate representation of ligament behavior in these models.

These findings highlight the need to address and incorporate the viscoelastic properties of ligaments in computational models. By considering the time-dependent response and realistic viscoelastic behavior of ligaments, the accuracy and reliability of the models can be improved. Future research should focus on accurately characterizing and including ligament viscoelasticity in computational models to advance our understanding of ligament function and contribute to more effective injury prevention and rehabilitation strategies.

3.3.4. *Mechanical properties limitations*

Studies have investigated the fluid flow occurring inside ligaments to gain insights into their characteristics and properties. Through these investigations, it has been identified that certain parameters, such as the values of Poisson's ratio and shear properties, play a significant role in influencing fluid flow dynamics (Adceb *et al.*, 2004). It is crucial to carefully evaluate these variables, as they can have a substantial impact on the behavior of fluid flow within ligaments. By considering and properly assessing these parameters, a better understanding of the fluid flow phenomenon can be achieved, leading to improved insights into the biomechanics and functionality of ligaments.

As previously mentioned, various models used to study ligaments are subject to certain limitations that can impact the accuracy of the results. Here are some examples of these limitations:

- In several models, the consideration of ligament thickness is often overlooked, which can affect the representation of ligament behavior (Rahman *et al.*, 2016).

- Mathematical models tend to oversimplify the histology of ligaments, neglecting important anatomical details (Barrett and Callaghan, 2018).
- Finite element models commonly ignore the laxity of ligaments and assume them to be incompressible and hyperplastic, despite the fact that ligaments are actually compressible and viscoelastic structures (Lasswell *et al.*, 2017; Seo *et al.*, 2012).
- Constitutive models incorporate hyperplastic functions to better fit the mechanical response of ligaments. However, these models often neglect time-dependent effects such as viscoelasticity and strain rate, which are important for capturing the dynamic behavior of ligaments (Nikolopoulos *et al.*, 2012; Luetkemeyer *et al.*, 2021). Ligaments exhibit different mechanical responses under quasi-static and dynamic loads, necessitating accurate material property selection to represent their behavior in both scenarios (Davis and De Vita, 2014; Kernozek and Ragan, 2008).
- Musculoskeletal models make assumptions of static equilibrium in the knee-ligament loading, disregarding the effects of centrifugal and inertial forces, which can impact the accuracy of the results (Shelburne *et al.*, 2004).
- Mechanistic modeling assumes that each collagen fiber within ligaments independently generates force linearly, overlooking the complex interplay and non-linear behavior of these fibers (Barrett and Callaghan, 2017).

3.3.5. *Material properties limitations*

The characterization of ligament materials in models presents significant challenges due to their inherent complexity (Jiang *et al.*, 2015). One specific limitation is the unavailability of stiffness properties for certain ligaments, which necessitates extrapolation and introduces potential errors in the simulations (Haraguchi *et al.*, 2009). These material property limitations highlight the difficulty in accurately representing the complex behavior of ligaments in computational models. Further research and advancements are needed to improve the characterization and incorporation of material properties in order to enhance the accuracy and reliability of ligament simulations.

These limitations highlight the challenges in accurately representing the intricate behavior of ligaments within different modeling approaches. Addressing these limitations and incorporating more comprehensive and realistic representations of ligament properties and behavior will be crucial for advancing our understanding of ligament biomechanics.

3.3.6. *Model-specific limitations*

Finite element models are commonly employed to study ligaments, either by modeling the entire knee joint or focusing specifically on the ligament itself. Both approaches facilitate the analysis of ligament stresses, strains, insertion site forces, and load transfer to bones through contact, while the full joint model additionally allows for the evaluation of joint kinematics. Laser scanning and medical imaging are the two primary techniques used to generate the geometry of ligaments.

Laser scanning offers high accuracy but lacks the ability to distinguish between the ligament of interest and surrounding bone and soft tissue structures. On the other hand, medical imaging techniques can provide more comprehensive information but may have lower geometric accuracy. Constitutive equations are commonly employed to describe the behavior of ligament materials within these models. However, it is important to note that no finite element model can be fully validated or verified, indicating the inherent limitations in achieving a perfect representation (Weiss and Gardiner, 2001).

These model-specific limitations highlight the challenges in accurately capturing the complexity of ligament behavior and geometry within finite element models. Ongoing research and advancements are necessary to improve the accuracy, validation, and verification of these models to enhance our understanding of ligament mechanics and their role in joint function.

3.3.7. *Medical imaging limitations*

Localization of ligament insertion sites in magnetic resonance imaging (MRI) scans is typically achieved using defined points, which provide information about the ligament's attachment points (Innocenti *et al.*, 2016; Smale *et al.*, 2019). While defining an area can be beneficial for clinical and biomechanical purposes, MRI scans have limitations in displaying the ligaments in three dimensions (Innocenti *et al.*, 2016). Despite being considered the standard for knee structure visualization, no reports have indicated that MRI scans can accurately depict ligaments in detail in three dimensions. In contrast, dual-energy computerized tomography (DECT) scans have been investigated as an alternative method capable of producing multi-angled images of ligaments. However, these scans have limitations in displaying thinner and transverse ligaments satisfactorily, and the scanning time required is two–three times longer (Sun *et al.*, 2008). This limitation hinders the widespread use of dual-energy CT images for ligament visualization.

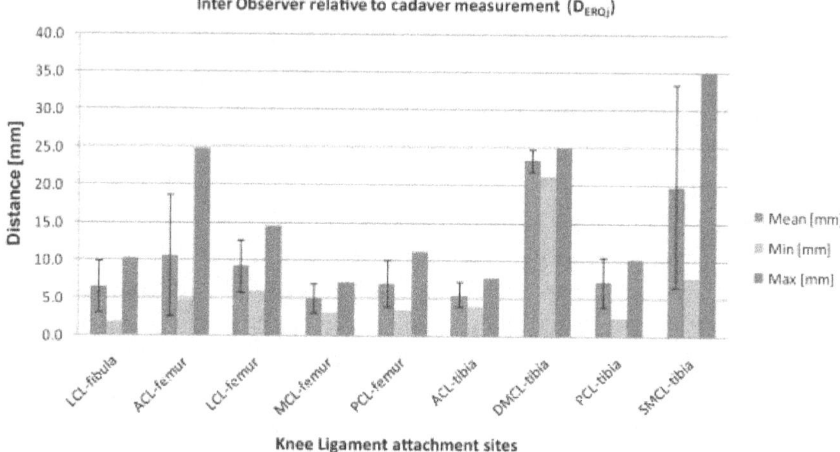

Fig. 3.   Variabilities of distances of the ligaments' attachment sites relative to the point position of physical cadaver measurements for inter-observation.
Source: Rachmat *et al.* (2014).

Moreover, there can be significant variations in identifying the attachment sites of knee ligaments from MRI scans. Certain ligament attachment sites, such as the deep and superficial medial collateral ligament (MCL) insertion, are particularly challenging to replicate accurately, with an average error of up to 23.39 mm which is shown in Fig. 3 (Rachmat *et al.*, 2014).

These limitations in ligament visualization using MRI and dual-energy CT scans underscore the need for further advancements in imaging techniques to improve the accurate representation and characterization of ligament structures.

4. Discussion

The studies on computational modeling of ligaments have identified several limitations that affect the accuracy and comprehensiveness of these models. Some of the limitations include the following:

(1) Inaccurate insertion sites: The exact attachment points of ligaments are challenging to determine accurately, and this uncertainty can introduce errors in the models.

(2) Ignoring viscoelasticity: Ligaments exhibit time-dependent behavior, meaning their mechanical properties change over time. Many models overlook this viscoelastic nature, which can affect the accuracy of predictions.

(3) Overlooking zero-load length parameter: Ligaments have a characteristic length at which they exert minimal force, known as the zero-load length. Neglecting this parameter can lead to inaccurate representation of ligament behavior.
(4) Straight-line approximation: Some models simplify ligaments by assuming they are straight lines, which does not accurately capture their complex three-dimensional structure.
(5) Disregarding time-dependent effects: Time-dependent effects, such as creep and stress relaxation, are important in ligament mechanics. However, many models do not account for these phenomena.

While there are other limitations, the ones mentioned above are considered particularly significant in terms of inducing errors in the computational models. Ligaments possess a range of complex characteristics that make their accurate modeling challenging. They are nonlinear (their behavior is not proportional to the applied load), anisotropic (their mechanical properties vary with direction), viscoelastic (their response depends on the rate of loading), and inhomogeneous (their properties vary within their structure). Despite these limitations, limited computational models have demonstrated the ability to produce accurate results. However, these models often lack the inclusion of extrinsic factors such as time and physiological effects like muscle atrophy. Future research in this field can focus on improving computational modeling of ligaments by incorporating all the structural characteristics discussed above, as well as considering the influence of extrinsic factors.

By including intrinsic factors and accounting for extrinsic factors, such as time and physiological effects, more advanced computational models of ligaments can be developed. This would lead to significant advancements in the field of biomechanics, enhancing our understanding of ligament function, injury mechanisms, and rehabilitation strategies.

Indeed, as models continue to advance, it becomes increasingly important to simulate the changes in the structure and function of ligaments over time, as well as their response to environmental hazards. These simulations can provide valuable insights into the behavior of ligaments under different conditions and help researchers and clinicians better understand how they adapt and respond to various factors.

Time-dependent effects play a crucial role in ligament mechanics, and incorporating them into computational models can provide a more accurate representation of ligament behavior. By considering the time-dependent properties of ligaments, such as creep (the gradual deformation under constant load) and stress relaxation (the decrease in stress over time under constant strain), models can better predict the long-term behavior and response of ligaments.

Furthermore, environmental hazards and external factors can have a significant impact on ligament structure and function. For example, factors like mechanical loading, temperature variations, exposure to chemicals or toxins, and aging can influence the properties and behavior of ligaments. Including these environmental hazards in computational models allows for a more comprehensive understanding of ligament responses and can aid in the development of preventive strategies and rehabilitation protocols.

By integrating the effects of time and environmental hazards into computational models, researchers can simulate and study the dynamic changes in ligaments, providing a deeper understanding of their adaptation, degradation, and repair processes. This knowledge can have important implications in various fields, including biomechanics, sports science, orthopedics, and tissue engineering, enabling the development of improved preventive measures, treatment strategies, and rehabilitation protocols for ligament-related injuries and conditions.

Funding

None

Conflict of Interest

There is no conflict of interest in this project.

Data Availability

All data, detailed in Appendix C, can be accessed through any journal database or Google Scholar.

References

Adeeb, S, Ali, A, Shrive, N, Frank, CY and Smith, D (2004) Modeling the behavior of ligaments: A technical note, *Comput. Methods Biomech. Biomed. Eng.* **7**(1), 33–42.

Aromataris, E *et al.* (2015) Summarizing systematic reviews: Methodological development, conduct and reporting of an umbrella review approach, *Int. J. Evid. Based Healthc.* **13**(3), 132–140.

Baldwin, MA, Clary, CW, Fitzpatrick, CK, Deacy, JS, Maletsky, LP and Rullkoetter, PJ (2012) Dynamic finite element knee simulation for evaluation of knee replacement mechanics, *J. Biomech.* **45**(3), 474–483.

Barrett, JM and Callaghan, JP (2017) A mechanistic damage model for ligaments, *J. Biomech.* **61**, 11–17.

Barrett, JM and Callaghan, JP (2018) A procedure for determining parameters of a simplified ligament model, *J. Biomech.* **66**, 175–179.

Blemker, SS *et al.* (2007) Image-based musculoskeletal modeling: Applications, advances, and future opportunities, *J. Magn. Reson. Imaging* **25**(2), 441–451.

Carey, RE *et al.* (2014) Subject-specific finite element modeling of the tibiofemoral joint based on CT, magnetic resonance imaging and dynamic stereo-radiography data *in vivo*, *J. Biomech. Eng.* **136**(4), 041004.

Davis, FM and De Vita, R (2014) A three-dimensional constitutive model for the stress relaxation of articular ligaments, *Biomech. Model. Mechanobiol.* **13**(3), 653–663.

Dhillon, MS, Bali, K and Prabhakar, S (2012) Differences among mechanoreceptors in healthy and injured anterior cruciate ligaments and their clinical importance, *Muscles Liagaments Tendons J.* **2**(1), 38–43.

Di Gregorio, R *et al.* (2007) Mathematical models of passive motion at the human ankle joint by equivalent spatial parallel mechanisms, *Med. Biol. Eng. Comput.* **45**(3), 305–313.

Farrell, PSE (1999) The hysteresis effect, *Hum. Factors* **41**(2), 226–240.

Frank, CB (2004) Ligament structure, physiology and function, *J. Musculoskelet. Neuronal Interact.* **4**(2), 199–201.

Hamidrad, S, Abdollahi, M, Badali, V, Nikkhoo, M and Naserkhaki, S (2021) Biomechanical modeling of spinal ligaments: Finite element analysis of L4-L5 spinal segment, *Comput. Methods Biomech. Biomed. Eng.* **24**(16), 1807–1818.

Haraguchi, N, Armiger, RS, Myerson, MS, Campbell, JT and Chao, EYS (2009) Prediction of three-dimensional contact stress and ligament tension in the ankle during stance determined from computational modeling, *Foot Ankle Int.* **30**(2), 177–185.

Innocenti, B, Salandra, P, Pascale, W and Pianigiani, S (2016) How accurate and reproducible are the identification of cruciate and collateral ligament insertions using MRI? *Knee* **23**(4), 575–581.

Jiang, Y, Wang, Y and Peng, X (2015) A visco-hyperelastic constitutive model for human spine ligaments, *Cell Biochem. Biophys.* **71**(2), 1147–1156.

Jung, H-J, Fisher, MB and Woo, SLY (2009) Role of biomechanics in the understanding of normal, injured, and healing ligaments and tendons, *BMC Sports Sci. Med. Rehabil.* **1**(1), 9.

Kazemi, M, Dabiri, Y and Li, LP (2013) Recent advances in computational mechanics of the human knee joint, *Comput. Math. Methods Med.* **2013**, 718423.

Kernozek, TW and Ragan, RJ (2008) Estimation of anterior cruciate ligament tension from inverse dynamics data and electromyography in females during drop landing, *Clin. Biomech. (Bristol, Avon)* **23**(10), 1279–1286.

Kim, YH, Khuyagbaatar, B and Kim, K (2018) Recent advances in finite element modeling of the human cervical spine, *J. Mech. Sci. Technol.* **32**(1), 1–10.

Lasswell, TL *et al.* (2017) Incorporating ligament laxity in a finite element model for the upper cervical spine, *Spine J.* **17**(11), 1755–1764.

Lim, Y *et al.* (2022) Challenges in kinetic-kinematic driven musculoskeletal subject-specific infant modeling, *Math. Comput. Appl.* **27**, 36, doi:10.3390/mca27030036.

Luetkemeyer, CM, Scheven, U, Estrada, JB and Arruda, EM (2021) Constitutive modeling of the anterior cruciate ligament bundles and patellar tendon with full-field methods, *J. Mech. Phys. Solids* **156**, 104577.

Marra, MA *et al.* (2015) A subject-specific musculoskeletal modeling framework to predict *in vivo* mechanics of total knee arthroplasty, *J. Biomech. Eng.* **137**(2), 020904.

Mierke, CT (2021) Viscoelasticity acts as a marker for tumor extracellular matrix characteristics, *Front. Cell Dev. Biol.* **9**, 785138.

Nikolopoulos, FV, Poulilios, AD, Stamou, AC, Papagelopoulos, PJ, Zoubos, AV and Kefalas, VA (2012) A simple constitutive model for the Scapholunate ligament, *Med. Eng. Phys.* **34**(8), 1196–1199.

Page, MJ *et al.* (2021) The PRISMA 2020 statement: An updated guideline for reporting systematic reviews. *BMJ* **372**, n71.

Peel, SA *et al.* (2023) Knee joint function in healthy and ACL-reconstructed collegiate female lacrosse players: A pilot study, *J. Sci. Sport Exerc.*, doi:10.1007/s42978-023-00223-2.

Peters, AE *et al.* (2018) Tissue material properties and computational modeling of the human tibiofemoral joint: A critical review, *PeerJ* **6**, e4298.

Rachmat, HH *et al.* (2014) Generating finite element models of the knee: How accurately can we determine ligament attachment sites from MRI scans? *Med. Eng. Phys.* **36**(6), 701–707.

Rahman, M, Cil, A, Bogener, JW and Stylianou, AP (2016) Lateral collateral ligament deficiency of the elbow joint: A modeling approach, *J. Orthop. Res.* **34**(9), 1645–1655.

Screen, HRC (2008) Investigating load relaxation mechanics in tendon, *J. Mech. Behav. Biomed. Mater.* **1**(1), 51–58.

Seo, Y-J, Yoo, Y-S, Noh, K-C, Song, S-Y, Lee, Y-B, Kim, H-J and Kim, HY (2012) Dynamic function of coracoclavicular ligament at different shoulder abduction angles: A study using a 3-dimensional finite element model, *Arthroscopy* **28**(6), 778–787.

Shelburne, KB, Pandy, MG, Anderson, FC and Torry, MR (2004) Pattern of anterior cruciate ligament force in normal walking, *J. Biomech.* **37**(6), 797–805.

Shelburne, KB and Pandy, MG (1997) A musculoskeletal model of the knee for evaluating ligament forces during isometric contractions, *J. Biomech.* **30**(2), 163–176.

Smale, KB, Conconi, M, Sancisi, N, Krogsgaard, M, Alkjaer, T, Parenti-Castelli, V and Benoit, DL (2019) Effect of implementing magnetic resonance imaging for patient-specific OpenSim models on lower-body kinematics and knee ligament lengths, *J. Biomech.* **83**, 9–15.

Solomonow, M (2009) Ligaments: A source of musculoskeletal disorders, *J. Bodyw. Mov. Ther.* **13**(2), 136–154.

Sun, C, Miao, F, Wang, X-M, Wang, T, Ma, R, Wang, D-P and Liu, C (2008) An initial qualitative study of dual-energy CT in the knee ligaments, *Surg. Radiol. Anat.* **30**(5), 443–447.

Tian, R *et al.* (2010) A multiresolution continuum simulation of the ductile fracture process, *J. Mech. Phys. Solids* **58**(10), 1681–1700.

Vanness, DJ *et al.* (2005) The need for microsimulation to evaluate osteoporosis interventions, *Osteoporos. Int.* **16**(4), 353–358.

Walck, CD (2019) *Biomechanical Response of the Knee Complex to a Non-Linear Spring-Loaded Knee Joint Orthosis*, PhD thesis, Embry-Riddle Aeronautical University, Ann Arbor.

Weiss, JA and Gardiner, JC (2001) Computational modeling of ligament mechanics, *Crit. Rev. Biomed. Eng.* **29**(3), 303–371.

Willemink, MJ *et al.* (2020) Preparing medical imaging data for machine learning, *Radiology* **295**(1), 4–15.

Yang, Z, Wickwire, AC and Debski, RE (2010) Development of a subject-specific model to predict the forces in the knee ligaments at high flexion angles, *Med. Biol. Eng. Comput.* **48**(11), 1077–1085.

Zhang, M, Davies, TC, Zhang, Y and Xie, SQ (2016) A real-time computational model for estimating kinematics of ankle ligaments, *Comput. Methods Biomech. Biomed. Eng.* **19**(8), 835–844.

Zhou, J *et al.* (2021) Tensile creep mechanical behavior of periodontal ligament: A hyper-viscoelastic constitutive model, *Comput. Methods Prog. Biomed.* **207**, 106224.

Appendix A. Search Strategy

Topic-specific search terms used in MEDLINE database:

(1) Ligament AND models;
(2) Ligament modeling;
(3) Ligament AND biomechanics;
(4) Modeling of ligaments.

Appendix B. Studies Excluded on Full Text

Ali, N, Anderson, MS, Rasmussen, J, Robertson, DGE and Rouhi, G (2014) The application of musculoskeletal modeling to investigate gender bias in non-contact ACL injury rate during single-leg landings, *Comput. Methods Biomech. Biomed. Eng.* **17**(14), 1602–1616.

Reason for exclusion: Did not include the description of ligament models.

Ancillao, A, Tedesco, S, Barton, J and O'Flynn, B (2018) Indirect measurement of ground reaction forces and moments by means of wearable inertial sensors: A systematic review, *Sensors (Basel)* **18**(8), 2564.

Reason for exclusion: Did not include the description of ligament model limitations.

Pollard, CD, Sigward, SM and Powers, CM (2017) ACL injury prevention training results in modification of hip and knee mechanics during a drop-landing task, *Orthop. J. Sports Med.* **5**(9), 2325967117726267.

Reason for exclusion: Did not include the ligament models.

Trickey, EL (1976) Ligamentous injuries around the knee, *Br. Med. J.* **2**(6050), 1492–1494.

Reason for exclusion: Did not include the ligament models.
Galbusera, F, Cina, A, Panico, M, Albano, D and Messina, C (2020) Image-based biomechanical models of the musculoskeletal system, *Eur. Radiol. Exp.* **4**, 49.

Reason for exclusion: Did not include the description of ligament model limitations.
Galbusera, F, Cina, A, Panico, M, Albano, D and Messina, C (2020) Image-based biomechanical models of the musculoskeletal system, *Eur. Radiol. Exp.* **4**, 49.

Reason for exclusion: Did not include the ligament models.
Guess, TM, Razu, S and Jahandar, H (2016) Evaluation of knee ligament mechanics using computational models, *J. Knee Surg.* **29**(2), 126–137.

Reason for exclusion: Not peer-reviewed.
Hui, C, Yeli, P, Swami, V, Mabee, M and Jaremko, JL (2016) A validation study of a novel 3-dimensional MRI modeling technique to identify the anatomic insertions of the anterior cruciate ligament, *Orthop. J. Sports Med.* **4**(12), 2325967116673797.

Reason for exclusion: Did not include the ligament models.
Li, K, Du, J, Huang, L-X, Ni, L, Liu, T and Yang, H-L (2017) The diagnostic accuracy of magnetic resonance imaging for anterior cruciate ligament injury in comparison to arthroscopy: A meta-analysis, *Sci. Rep.* **7**(1), 7583.

Reason for exclusion: Did not include the ligament models.
Lee, M and Hyman, W (2002) Modeling of failure mode in knee ligaments depending on the strain rate, *BMC Musculoskelet. Disord.* **3**, 3.

Reason for exclusion: Did not include the ligament models.
Buckthorpe, M, Tamisari, A and Della Villa, F (2020) A ten task-based progression in rehabilitation after ACL reconstruction: from post-surgery to return to play — A clinical commentary, *Int. J. Sports Phys. Ther.* **15**(4), 611–623.

Reason for exclusion: Did not include the description of ligament model limitations.
Paxton, JZ, Donnelly, K, Keatch, RP, Baar, K and Grover, LM (2010) Factors affecting the longevity and strength in an *in vitro* model of the bone-ligament interface, *Ann. Biomed. J.* **38**(6), 2155–2166.

Reason for exclusion: Did not include the ligament models.
Readioff, R, Geraghty, B, Comerford, E and Elsheikh, A (2020) A full-field 3D digital image correlation and modeling technique to characterise anterior cruciate ligament mechanics *ex vivo*, *Acta Biomater.* **113**, 417–428.

Reason for exclusion: Did not include the ligament models.
Fickert, S, Niks, M, Dinter, DJ, Hammer, M, Weckbach, S, Schoenberg, SO, Lehmann, L and Jochum, S (2013) Assessment of the diagnostic value of dual-energy CT and MRI in the detection of iatrogenically induced injuries of anterior cruciate ligament in a porcine model, *Skeletal Radiol.* **42**(3), 411–417.

Reason for exclusion: Did not include the ligament models.
Trinler, U, Schwameder, H, Baker, R and Alexander, N (2019) Muscle force estimation in clinical gait analysis using AnyBody and OpenSim, *J. Biomech.* **86**, 55–63.

Reason for exclusion: Did not include the description of ligament model limitations.
Bousson, V, Lowitz, T, Laouisset, L, Engelke, K and Laredo, J-D (2012) CT imaging for the investigation of subchondral bone in knee osteoarthritis, *Osteoporos. Int.* **23**(Suppl. 8), S861–S865.

Reason for exclusion: Did not include the ligament models.
Pedoia, V, Lansdown, DA, Zaid, M, McCulloch, CE, Souza, R, Ma, CB and Li, X (2015) Three-dimensional MRI-based statistical shape model and application to a cohort of knees with acute ACL injury, *Osteoarthritis Cartilage* **23**(10), 1695–1703.

Reason for exclusion: Did not include the ligament models.
Herzog, W (1998) History dependence of force production in skeletal muscle: A proposal for mechanisms, *J. Electromyogr. Kinesiol.* **8**(2), 111–117.

Reason for exclusion: Did not include the ligament models.
Zheng, YP and Mak, AF (1999) Extraction of quasi-linear viscoelastic parameters for lower limb soft tissues from manual indentation experiment, *J. Biomech. Eng.* **121**(3), 330–339.

Reason for exclusion: Did not include the ligament models.

Appendix C. Characteristics of Included Studies

Table C.1.　Characteristics of included studies: Systematic review and research syntheses form.

Study	Review objectives	Descriptions of interventions/ phenomena of interest	Descriptions of outcomes included in the review	Descriptions of contexts included in the review	Description of main results
Woo, SL-Y, Johnson, GA and Smith, BA (1993)	This paper presents a survey of developments in mathematical modeling of ligaments and tendons over the past 20 years	Ligament and tendon properties and their behaviors	NA	Structural and phenomenological models, elastic models, and viscoelastic models	(i) Mathematical descriptions of ligaments and tendons are identified as either elastic or viscoelastic and are discussed in chronological order. (ii) Elastic models assume that ligaments and tendons do not display time-dependent behavior and thus, they focus on describing the nonlinear aspects of their mechanical response. (iii) On the other hand, viscoelastic models incorporate time-dependent effects into their mathematical description. In particular, two viscoelastic models are discussed in detail; quasi-linear viscoelasticity (QLV), which has been widely used in the past 20 years, and the recently proposed single integral finite strain (SIFS) model.

Table C.1.   (*Continued*)

Study	Review objectives	Descriptions of interventions/ phenomena of interest	Descriptions of outcomes included in the review	Descriptions of contexts included in the review	Description of main results
Fernandez, JW and Pandy, MG (2006)	This paper reviews these various technologies in the context of their application to the study of human movement. They describe how three-dimensional, subject-specific computer models of the muscles, ligaments, cartilage, and bones can be developed from high-resolution magnetic resonance images; how X-ray fluoroscopy can be used to measure the relative movements of the bones at a joint in three dimensions with submillimeter accuracy; how complex 3D dynamic simulations of movement can be performed using new computational methods based on nonlinear control theory; and how musculoskeletal forces derived from such simulations can be used as inputs to elaborate finite element models of a joint to calculate the contact stress distributions on a subject-specific basis	Intensive research has been carried out over the last 30 years to understand the conditions necessary for maintaining healthy cartilage and the mechanical and biochemical environment that leads to the disease. Much has been learnt about the morphology, biochemistry, and mechanics of cartilage, but many of the important questions remain unanswered. For example, what are the dynamic loading conditions to which cartilage is exposed during daily activity, and how does this environment influence the health of the tissue? The answers are fundamental for diagnosing and treating joint disease, since dynamic loading affects the movement of tissue growth factors, and tissue growth factors must be transported into the cartilage layer to keep it healthy. One key difficulty in understanding these issues has been the inability to measure bone movements accurately *in-vivo*	A hierarchical modeling approach is highlighted that links rigid-body models of limb segments with detailed finite element models of the joints. A framework is proposed that integrates subject-specific musculoskeletal computer models with highly accurate *in-vivo* experimental data	NA	The result would be contact loads and FE deformable body kinematics based on the applied muscle forces and ligament constraints. Most of the steps outlined in Fig. 7 have been previously developed by the authors. Methods related to X-ray imaging and the pose-estimation problem have been reported by others (Banks and Hodge, 1996; Fregly *et al.*, 2004; Li *et al.*, 2005). Their immediate goal is to integrate the various steps described above to produce a practical and economical diagnostic tool for noninvasively assessing musculoskeletal function on a subject-specific basis.

Table C.2.   Characteristics of included studies: Quasi-experimental study form.

Study	Country	Setting/context	Participant characteristics	Groups	Outcomes measured
Adeeb, S, Ali, A, Shrive, N, Frank, CY and Smith, D (2004)	Canada?	(i) Examining three different mechanisms of how fluid is exuded from ligaments subject to tensile loading. (1) Mechanism 1: Difference in volumes between barrel shapes and cylinders having equal edge lengths, which represent the crimp/curvature of initially unloaded ligaments. This mechanism is investigated with simple mathematical calculations of volumes. (2) Mechanism 2: Investigation through finite element modeling of the effect of having a high Poisson's ratio between the lateral and longitudinal directions, as recorded in the literature. (3) Mechanism 3: Examined with the finite element method, involving the effect of osmotic pressure, which would cause the unloaded ligament to swell and have an initial barrel shape	NA	How fluid is exuded from ligaments subject to tensile loading?	(i) Studies have shown that the fibers are initially "crimped", taking helical or waveform shapes. The straightening of the waveform shape is thought to be partly responsible for the existence of a "toe region" in the stress–strain curve of the tensile test of a ligament. Their first mechanism model is a simplification of the issue that a fiber is not likely to be straight between its insertion point on one bone and its insertion point on the other. (ii) Imposing horizontal and vertical restraints at the insertion site, as done here, is not an exact way of modeling the insertion site, because it does not allow for the possible fiber realignment at the insertion with the direction of loading. (iii) Limitations/gaps: (1) First, there is no change in permeability with voids ratio: strain-dependent changes in permeability occur in cartilage, so may also occur in ligaments. (2) The applied osmotic pressure was held constant on the free surface with no allowance for changes in ion concentration. (3) In the models for mechanisms 2 and 3, the fibers were assumed to lie directly between insertion points: no curved fibers were included in the finite element models. (iv) Thus, to model ligaments more exactly, and understand their behavior more clearly, several new parameters need to be investigated experimentally. Values of Poisson's ratio and shear properties need to be determined carefully as these parameters have a great effect on the fluid flow inside the ligament.

Table C.2.   (*Continued*)

Study	Country	Setting/context	Participant characteristics	Groups	Outcomes measured
Johnson, GA, Livesay, GA, Woo, SL and Rajagopal, KR (1996)	USA	(i) A general continuum model for the nonlinear viscoelastic behavior of soft biological tissues was formulated. (ii) This single integral finite strain model describes finite deformation of a nonlinearly viscoelastic material within the context of a three- dimensional model	NA	Predicting time-dependent stress generated by cyclic extensions	Work provided in this paper provides a theoretical framework and a specific model for ligaments and tendons undergoing uniaxial tension.
Debski, RE, Darcy, SP and Woo, SLY (2004)	USA	Quantitative data on the mechanics of diarthrodial joints and the function of ligaments are needed to better understand injury mechanisms, improve surgical procedures, and develop improved rehabilitation protocols. Therefore, experimental and computational approaches have been developed to determine joint kinematics and the *in-situ* forces in ligaments and their replacement grafts using human cadaveric knee and shoulder joints	NA	Experimental data used to validate computation models	(i) In the future, this combined approach will improve their understanding of these joints and soft tissues during *in-vivo* activities and serve as a tool in aiding surgical planning and development of rehabilitation protocols. (ii) These models can predict forces and strains in the ligaments at varying levels of daily activities and in response to rehabilitation protocols.

(*Continued*)

Table C.2. (*Continued*)

Study	Country	Setting/context	Participant characteristics	Groups	Outcomes measured
Weiss, JA and Gardiner, JC (2001)	USA	(i) Develop a framework for subject-specific modeling of ligament mechanics and to critically evaluate the effectiveness of the framework for predicting strain distributions in the loaded joint. (ii) Dissertation investigated the mechanics of the human medial collateral ligament and developed a number of tools that will facilitate future study of other ligaments and biological tissues	NA	NA	(i) Framework for parameter estimation will be used to develop new ligament constitutive models that will improve future finite element models. (ii) Currently developed modeling methodologies can ultimately assist with patient-specific surgical planning and education and to study the effects of tissue-level deformations on local cellular mechanotransduction.
Peña, E, Peña, JA and Doblaré, M (2008)	UK	The goal of this study is to characterize and demonstrate the importance of the nonlinear stress relaxation behavior of ligaments undergoing finite deformation	NA	Model that describes experimentally observed nonlinear viscoelastic behavior of soft tissues	(i) Model provides a very efficient tool to determine realistic predictions of stress, strain, and strain rate distributions in ligaments with different viscoelastic behaviors of collagen tissue and ground substance. (ii) Limitations: (1) Most remarkable is related with the QLV character of the formulation, so the model is restricted to small perturbations from equilibrium (Haslach, 2005). (2) Another remarkable limitation is the need of an elevated number of parameters: (a) In fact, a nonlinear viscoelastic model with internal variables is the minimum required. (b) However, this implies 20 material parameters (four for the hyperelastic part and 16 for the viscoelastic part). (3) Finally, the damage phenomena occurring in the connective tissue, which are a consequence of the application of nonphysiological loads or of degenerative processes, should be included in the formulation of the model as well. (4) In fact, the hyperelastic model with damage presented in Calvo *et al.* (2006) could be the basis for the development of a more general viscoelastic constitutive model (Peña *et al.*, 2008).

Table C.2.   (*Continued*)

Study	Country	Setting/context	Participant characteristics	Groups	Outcomes measured
Hamidrad, S, Abdollahi, M, Badali, V, Nikkhoo, M and Naserkhaki, S (2021)	UK?	(i) Different 3D models of L4–L5 spinal segment cistinguished by their ligament modeling were developed (1D truss, 2D shell, and 3D space truss elements). (ii) Aimed to develop a 3D model for the ligaments during different loading conditions	CT scans of healthy person	ROM, intra-discal pressure, and stress/force of ligament	(i) Limitations: (1) Ligament failure/injury mechanism was not simulated here: (a) Their main focus here was to investigate the effect of the ligament modeling in elastic range which kept the analysis in physiological range of motion without failure/injury occurrence. (2) Ligaments' viscoelastic property was ignored here since their immediate static behavior was concerned in this study. (3) Current model also overlooked ligament pre-straining in order to avoid any changes in model geometry. (4) Since this was a comparative study between different models (different ligament models), the ligament pre-straining could not present a major effect on the conclusion. (ii) Information would enhance their understanding about the potential locations of the failure/injury in spinal ligaments.
Kiapour, AM, Kaul, V, Kiapour, A, Quatman, CE, Wordeman, SC, Hewett, TE, Demetropoulos, CK and Goel, VK (2014)	USA	Purpose of this study was to determine the effect of two most common techniques utilized to model knee ligaments on joint kinematics under functional loading conditions	Computerized tomography and magnetic resonance imaging scans of a young adult female Athlete's lower limb (age: 25 years, height: 170 cm, weight: 64.4 kg)	Study the effects of soft tissue material models	(i) The 3D anisotropic hyperelastic model resulted in a more physiological prediction of the human knee motion under ranges of single- and multi-planar functional loading conditions with strong correlation and minimal deviation from experimental data. (ii) Lower correlations in addition to notable deviations were observed using simplified uniaxial modeling technique.

(*Continued*)

Table C.2.   (*Continued*)

Study	Country	Setting/context	Participant characteristics	Groups	Outcomes measured
Sancisi, N, Gasparutto, X, Parenti-Castelli, V and Dumas, R (2017)	The Nether-lands?	This study presents a mathematical framework to implement a kinematic model of the knee featuring articular contacts and ligaments in the multi- body optimization	NA	Deformable ligament constraints in joint kinematic models	(i) This approach appears to be a good compromise between standard nonphysiological kinematic models and complex deformable dynamic models. (ii) It should be noted that one of the main issues with the penalty method is the weight definition: (1) In this study, ligament weights are chosen upon qualitative assumptions based on the literature and on the *in-vitro* experimental data. (iii) The geometrical model is not personalized and the experimental ligament lengthening, used in particular for $\Delta L\vartheta$, was measured *in-vitro* during natural joint motion: (1) Personalization can actually improve the MBO efficiency for STA compensation (Weiss and Gardiner, 2001), but the experimental procedures can be more complicated since the model parameters have to be measured on a subject, and the computational burden for model definition increases.
Pflum, MA, Shelburne, KB, Torry, MR, Decker, MJ and Pandy, MG (2004)	USA	The aim of this study was to calculate and explain the pattern of force transmitted to the anterior cruciate ligament during soft-style drop-landings	Single subject	Angles, activations, and forces	(i) Limitations: (1) Analysis performed on one subject. (2) Optimization theory was not used to predict muscle coordination during simulated drop-landing maneuver. (3) Knee-ligament forces calculated assuming that lower leg remained in static equilibrium. (4) Calculation of ligament loading neglected axial rotation of bones at knee. (5) First peak in horizontal ground reaction force did not match the result obtained from experiment.

Table C.2.   (*Continued*)

Study	Country	Setting/context	Participant characteristics	Groups	Outcomes measured
Nie, B, Panzer, MB, Mane, A, Mait, AR, Donlon, J-P, Forman, JL and Kent, RW (2016)	USA	This study developed a framework to parameterize the ligament response for determining the *in-situ* stress state and heterogeneous force–elongation characteristics using a finite element ankle model	NA	Responses of ankle ligaments during gross foot and ankle motions	(i) Limitations: (1) Bi-linear force–elongation behavior was introduced in the fiber material model as a representative of its mechanical behavior. (2) Ligament geometry was defined according to the geometrical features of the ankle bones. (3) Further research efforts are necessary to quantify the potential influence on the ligament response due to the variability of the bone geometry. (4) The role of musculotendinous structures is important to the ankle joint stability since the muscle contraction may influence the ligament tension (Baumhauer *et al.*, 1995).
Kar, J and Quesada, PM (2013)	USA	The central goal of this study was to contribute to the advancements being made in determining the underlying causes of anterior cruciate ligament (ACL) injuries	Eleven female recreational athletes with an average body weight of 59.7 ± 7.7 kg (1 SD), a height of 164.4 ± 12.7 cm, and a median age of 20 years participated in stop-jump activities	This study investigated stop-jumps and factors related to ACL injury like knee valgus and internal–external (IE) moment loads, knee anterior–posterior (AP) shear forces, ACL strains, and internal forces	(i) Limitations: (1) Lack of EMG data from the remaining muscles which could have been used to simulate an EMG-driven stop-jump task. (2) Finding muscle activations using the excitation–activation relationship given in Eq. (1) where the other methods for decoupling joint loads exist. (3) Not attempting to estimate physiological tibiofemoral compressive joint reaction force by replacing the fictitious patellotibial joint in the current model with a patellofemoral one as done in a previous study. (4) Whether maximum activations could be produced by other dynamic activities such as sprinting, squat-jumping, and cycling, none of which were scheduled for this study. (5) Studies (Kernozek and Ragan, 2008) that have compared isometric versus dynamic methods of obtaining MVCs have found small differences in peak magnitudes. (6) Muscle activation for the non-EMG muscles could not be compared to patterns of EMG (excitation) from other studies, mainly due to differing trial conditions.

(*Continued*)

Table C.2.   (Continued)

Study	Country	Setting/context	Participant characteristics	Groups	Outcomes measured
Zarei, V, Liu, CJ, Claeson, AA, Akkin, T and Barocas, VH (2017)	USA	The aim of this study was to characterize and incorporate in-plane local fiber structure into a multi-scale finite element model to predict the mechanical response of the FCL during *in-vitro* mechanical tests, accounting for the heterogeneity in different scales	Six healthy L4–L5 cadaveric lumbar FCLs	(i) Entire-domain collagen fiber organization in the lumbar FCL was characterized by PS-OCT. (ii) Macroscale FCL behavior was compared to *in-vitro* experiments through construction of subject-specific multi-scale finite element models based on the structural data	(i) Limitations: (1) The most significant limitation is the relatively low depth of imaging. (2) An additional simplification was the assumption that fibers run nearly parallel to the sample's surface. (ii) In terms of gross force–displacement behavior, their image-based model resulted in unsatisfactory agreement for two of the samples. (iii) They observe that the lumbar FCL is a complex tissue with heterogeneous organization at multiple scales.
Moglo, KE and Shirazi-Adl, A (2003)	Canada	To investigate the extent of coupling between the anterior and posterior cruciate ligaments as well as the role of the posterior cruciate ligament in the knee-joint response under anterior femoral force at different flexion angles	NA	To investigate the response of the fully unconstrained joint under 100-N femoral anterior force at different flexion angles	(i) Joint capsule was not modeled in this study. (ii) Remarkable novel coupling was noted in fully unconstrained flexion between cruciate ligaments in which PCL and ACL forces changed in tandem.
Salathe, EP and Arangio, GA (2002)	USA	Biomechanical model of the foot is developed and analyzed to determine the distribution of support under the metatarsal heads, the tension in the plantar aponeurosis, and the bending moment at each of the joints of the foot	NA	Distribution of support under the metatarsal heads, the tension in the plantar aponeurosis, and the bending moment at each of the joints of the foot	(i) Action of the muscles changes the support distribution among the metatarsal heads, and decreases the tension in the plantar aponeurosis and long plantar ligament, particularly the portions extending to the medial rays. (ii) Role of the intrinsic muscles has not been included in this model.

Table C.2.   (*Continued*)

Study	Country	Setting/context	Participant characteristics	Groups	Outcomes measured
Vaughan, N, Dubey, VN, Wee, MYK and Isaacs, R (2014)	UK	This work is to build upon the concept of matching a person's weight, height, and age to their overall body shape to create an adjustable three-dimensional model	For each patient, a set of standard anthropometric measurements are taken. These measurements are the inputs to the mathematical model: m (body mass, kg), h (height, cm), including a (age, years) and s (sex, male/female). Also, a qualitative description of body shape (Apple, Pear, Hourglass, or Banana) and the number of weeks pregnant are taken if applicable. These are chosen because they are easily achievable yet descriptive anthropometric data	(i) Three methods are provided for estimating body circumferences and ligament thicknesses for each patient: (1) First method is using empirical relations from body shape and size; (2) second method is to load a dataset from an MRI scan or ultrasound scan containing accurate ligament measurements; and (3) third method is the developed artificial neural network (ANN) which uses MRI dataset as a training set and improves accuracy using error back-propagation, which learns to increase accuracy as more patient data is added	(i) The quality criterion for skin and ligament thickness modeling was initially to produce results with higher accuracy: (1) Achieved results from ANN have accuracy within 3.54 mm, sufficient to produce a model of ligament thickness for epidural simulation with regard to training needs and the needs for implementing the approaches for clinical environments. (2) Advantages of the model include visualization of a general representation of external visual body shape and ability to adjust ligament thicknesses to match specific patients which may be useful for simulating intricate clinical procedures like epidurals.

(*Continued*)

Table C.2.   (*Continued*)

Study	Country	Setting/context	Participant characteristics	Groups	Outcomes measured
Zhang, M, Davies, TC, Zhang, Y and Xie, SQ (2016)	New Zealand	Ankle computational model was proposed and validated to quantify the kinematics of ankle ligaments as the foot moves in real-time	NA	Model uses inputs for three position variables that can be measured from sensors in many ankle robotic devices that detect postures within the foot–ankle environment and outputs the kinematics of ankle ligaments	(i) Model based on ligament lengths and strains is in concurrence with those from the published studies but is sensitive to ligament attachment positions. (ii) Limitations: (1) Bone geometry in this study was based on a generic ankle–foot complex model of LEM: (a) Scaling based on this generic model for subject-specific adaptation would contribute to improve the simulation precision. (2) Effects of the fusion of the tibia and fibula were unknown in this study. (3) Ligaments being represented as straight lines between origin and insertion points also introduce some simulation errors: (a) Origins and insertion points of these included ligaments were specified based on published anatomical data, and the model precision could be improved with subject-specific ligament locations by image-based methods such as MRI.

Table C.2.   (*Continued*)

Study	Country	Setting/context	Participant characteristics	Groups	Outcomes measured
Rahman, M, Cil, A, Bogener, JW and Stylianou, AP (2016)	USA	Purpose of this study was to simulate lateral collateral ligament deficiency during passive flexion using a computational multi-body elbow joint model and investigate the effects of ligament insufficiency on the kinematics, ligament loads, and articular contact characteristics (area, pressure)	A previously developed anatomically correct computational multi-body model created from a cadaver sample (61 years, male, right arm) was used as the basis	Four different conditions were simulated for this study: (i) simulation with all ligaments intact (baseline), (ii) simulation for RCL deficiency (Vanness *et al.*, 2005), (iii) simulation for LUCL deficiency, and (iv) simulation for combined RCL and LUCL deficiency	(i) Limitations: (1) Model is based on a single cadaver specimen and therefore characteristic of a single elbow: (a) Ligament deficiencies investigated here can give them insight into the role of the lateral complex in elbow stability but experimental validation studies involving larger sample sizes are required to generalize the conclusions. (2) The discretized cartilage parameters and discrete cartilage size were not optimized for this model but estimated using elastic foundation theory: (a) Future studies will optimize contact parameters and discretized cartilage size by matching the multi-body cartilage model to a finite element model. (3) The joint capsule works as a secondary static elbow stabilizer and the greatest contribution occurs with the elbow extended: (a) Their model did not incorporate the joint capsule contribution to joint stability and that may be one of the reasons for the slightly higher laxity observed in their results. (4) Their model did not employ muscles or fascia, so the stabilizing influence of these muscle tissues was not quantified in this study. (5) Since the ligaments are modeled as force elements, the thickness of the ligaments is not taken into account.

(*Continued*)

Table C.2.   (*Continued*)

Study	Country	Setting/context	Participant characteristics	Groups	Outcomes measured
Roux, A, Laporte, S, Lecompte, J, Gras, L-L and Iordanoff, I (2016)	France	Aims of this study were to model the MTC in DEM at the macroscopic scale and to obtain the force–displacement curve during a nondestructive passive tensile test	NA	The first step is to model MTC's tear. The aims of this study were to model the MTC using DEM, at a macroscopic scale, to reproduce the nonlinear force–displacement curve obtained experimentally for the passive muscle behavior during a nondestructive passive tensile test, and to highlight the influence of geometrical parameters of the MTC on the global mechanical behavior during a passive tensile test	Hyperelastic behavior of the stretching MTC was in agreement with *in-vitro* data. Geometry had a significant effect on the MTC's mechanical behavior. (iii) When the muscle's cross-sectional area increases, there is a tendency for the stress to decrease. (iv) When the muscle's cross-sectional area increases, there is a tendency for the stress to decrease. (v) Shape of numerical curve was in agreement with the curves obtained experimentally, confirming the possibility of modeling the nonlinear, hyperelastic macroscopic response of a muscle with simple, linear, elastic, microscopic elements.
Nikolopoulos, FV, Poulilios, AD, Stamou, AC, Papagelopoulos, PJ, Zoubos, AV and Kefalas, VA (2012)	Greece	A simple constitutive equation is presented to describe the nonlinear load–displacement behavior of the Scapholunate ligament (SL)	Specimens were harvested from five fresh cadaver forearm-wrists	Model was fitted to experimental results for the SL	(i) Time-dependent effects, including viscoelasticity, strain rate, etc., were ignored as second-order effects. (ii) Success of this simple three-constant model as a mathematical description implies that the assumption of structural molecular mechanism seems to be basically correct. (iii) The problem of homogeneity in living tissues is that selecting small specimens could lead to big miscalculations, because the selected specimens are not representative of the material of the overall tissue.

Table C.2.   (*Continued*)

Study	Country	Setting/context	Participant characteristics	Groups	Outcomes measured
Shelburne, KB, Pandy, MG, Anderson, FC and Torry, MR (2004)	USA	The goal of this study was to calculate and explain the pattern of anterior cruciate ligament loading during normal-level walking	Five subjects	Patterns of ACL loading during walking	(i) Limitations: (1) Assumption of static equilibrium in the calculation of knee-ligament loading, wherein the effects of centrifugal (velocity-dependent) and inertial forces were neglected. (2) Predictions of knee-ligament loading were also compromised by the fact that the dynamic optimization solution for walking was not fully converged. (3) Discontinuity in Vasti muscle force at contralateral toe-off obtained from the walking simulation led to a discontinuity in ACL force at contralateral toe-off.
Moissenet, F, Chèze, L and Dumas, R (2014)	Luxembourg, France	This study introduced a new 3D lower limb musculoskeletal model based on a one-step static optimization procedure allowing simultaneous musculotendon, joint contact, ligament, and bone forces estimation during gait	NA	Musculotendon forces, joint contact, ligament, and bone forces	(i) Models have been developed based on *in-vitro* unloaded knee movements and consider ligaments as isometric structures: (1) However, it has been shown that the kinematics of tibiofemoral and patellofemoral joints are similar between loaded and unloaded conditions during knee extension and that the ligament lengthening is limited during gait. (ii) Nevertheless, the isometric condition would have resulted in pushing ligaments (i.e. negative force) if the associated Lagrange multiplier has not been introduced in the optimization procedure: (1) This issue has been previously reported for the MCL force and can be avoided by introducing deformable ligaments in their model.

(*Continued*)

Table C.2.   (*Continued*)

Study	Country	Setting/context	Participant characteristics	Groups	Outcomes measured
Nie, B, Forman, JL, Panzer, MB, Mait, AR, Donlon, J-P and Kent, RW (2017)	USA	A fiber-based modeling approach of *in-situ* ankle ligaments was developed and validated for determining the heterogeneous force–elongation characteristics and the consequent injury patterns	Foot and ankle model, representing a mid-sized adult male foot, was used to functionally build up the ligamentous structures	Bony kinematics under foot rotation was replicated	(i) Model proved capable of predicting the bony motion under well-controlled external foot rotation from a parallel cadaveric study. (ii) The computational approach provided a useful tool for representing the mechanical properties of ligaments and the consequent joint mechanics at the structural level. (iii) The behaviors are consistent with the field observation that ankle ligament injury has a progressive nature, with the initial tear occurring at the border, growing to a complete rupture, and gradually reducing the sustained load down to zero. (iv) Limitations: (1) Viscoelastic and nonlinear behaviors of human ligaments, for either the midsubstance or the insertion site, were not considered. (2) Limited in the ability to represent the fiber-to-fiber interactions or nonhomogeneous strain distribution along the longitudinal axis in individual fiber bundles. (3) Foot geometry was anatomically reasonable and the experimental data were also limited to the specimens.
Pandy, MG, Sasaki, K and Kim, S (1997)	USA	Three-dimensional model of the knee is developed to study the interactions between the muscles, ligaments, and bones during activity	NA	Interactions between the muscles, ligaments, and bones	(i) Limitations: (1) Does not take into account inertial properties of leg. (2) Model assumes that the patellar tendon is inextensible. (3) Real ligaments attach over a finite area of bone and wrap around the bones and other ligaments during flexion.

Table C.2.   (*Continued*)

Study	Country	Setting/context	Participant characteristics	Groups	Outcomes measured
Shelburne, KB and Pandy, MG (1997)	USA	Model of the knee in the sagittal plane was developed to study the forces in the ligaments induced by isometric contractions of the extensor and flexor muscles	Twenty-three cadaveric knees	Ligament forces by isolated contractions of extensor and flexor muscles	(i) Limitations: (1) Model of knee is 2D. (2) Model assumes the length of the patellar ligament is constant over the entire range of knee flexions. (ii) Most significant contribution of the model is that it takes into account the effects of musculotendon properties and musculoskeletal geometry on calculations of cruciate ligament loading at the knee.
Lasswell, TL, Cronin, DS, Medley, JB and Rasoulinejad, P (2017)	Canada	Purpose of this study is to propose an optimization process that can be used to determine a set of ligament laxity values for upper cervical spine FE models	NA	Adapt this FE model to ROM scenarios of typical daily activities	(i) FE model (which included ligament laxity) was able to predict ROM data for upper cervical spine motions under axial rotation, flexion–extension, and lateral bending that was in good general agreement with experimental data. (ii) Limitations: (1) Anatomy of the FE model was generated from a single 50th percentile male. (2) Optimization study looked only at ligament laxities as varying inputs. (3) The anatomical geometry also plays a role in the ROM of the upper cervical spine, and this geometry is expected to change depending on gender, age, and stature. (4) The effect that anatomical geometry has on ligament laxity needs to be examined in future studies so that it can be included in the FE modeling approach. (5) All of the ligaments in the upper cervical spine were likely to have some laxity, and so the FE model was limited by only applying laxity to select ligaments.

(*Continued*)

Table C.2.   (*Continued*)

Study	Country	Setting/context	Participant characteristics	Groups	Outcomes measured
Gei, M, Genna, F and Bigoni, D (2002)	Italy	Nonlinear interface constitutive law is formulated for modeling the mechanical behavior of the periodontal ligament	NA	Effect of nonlinear behavior of PDL on the stress and strain states in the surrounding teeth and bone	(i) The nonlinear behavior of PDL produces extremely important effects on the computed mechanical quantities in a numerical model of the tooth-bone system. (ii) There are clear theoretical and computational advantages in employing an interface model in the numerical analyses, rather than a continuum, three-dimensional one. (iii) Difficulties: (1) The irreversibility of the PDL behavior, dominated by the presence and motion of the fluid phase, governed by its saturation index. (2) The fiber contents of PDL, as well as the position, orientation, geometry, and stiffness of the fibers.
Francis, WL, Eliason, TD, Thacker, BH, Paskoff, GR, Shender, BS and Nicolella, DP (2014)	USA	Objective of this investigation was to develop probabilistic FE models of the anterior longitudinal ligament (ALL) and posterior longitudinal ligament (PLL) of the cervical spine that incorporate the natural variability of biological specimens	NA	Dynamic stress–strain behaviors of PLL and ALL	(i) Able to fit a viscoelastic material model to dynamic relaxation experiments and test that model against dynamic tension–tension loading. (ii) Although many researchers have created ligament and spine models to predict mean responses, none are incorporating the actual large variations in material properties derived from experimental studies designed to calibrate and then validate biological material constitutive models: (1) By using a probabilistic model, the researcher can express response predictions in terms of probabilities.

Table C.2. (*Continued*)

Study	Country	Setting/context	Participant characteristics	Groups	Outcomes measured
Forestiero, A, Carniel, EL and Natali, AN (2014)	Italy	This study was aimed at the definition of a constitutive formulation of ankle ligaments and of a procedure for the constitutive parameters evaluation. for the biomechanical analysis by means of numerical models	Fresh cadaveric human ankles	Numerical model is provided for each experimental test developed	(i) A fiber-reinforced visco-hyperelastic constitutive model is developed to interpret the mechanical response of the ankle ligaments: (1) In agreement with experimental evidence, the constitutive formulation is capable of accounting for the typical features of ligament tissue mechanical behavior, such as the anisotropic configuration, nonlinear elasticity, and time-dependent phenomena.
Abdel-Rahman, EM and Hefzy, MS (1998)	USA, Saudi Arabia	The objective of this study is to determine the three-dimensional dynamic response of the human knee joint	This experimental study uses data from other studies	Knee response was studied by considering sudden external forcing pulse loads applied to the tibia	(i) Ligament wrapping was not taken into consideration. (ii) It is hard to validate this model's predictions because of the limited amount of experimental data available in the literature that describes the dynamic behavior of the human knee joint.
Davis, FM and De Vita, R (2014)	USA	(i) A new nonlinear constitutive model for the three-dimensional stress relaxation of articular ligaments is proposed. (ii) The model accounts for finite strains, anisotropy, and strain-dependent stress relaxation behavior exhibited by these ligaments. (iii) Direct comparison with stress relaxation data collected by subjecting human MCLs to shear deformation in the fiber direction is presented in order to demonstrate the predictive capabilities of the model	This model uses other studies' subject parameters	Direct comparison with stress relaxation data collected by subjecting human MCLs to shear deformation in the fiber direction is presented in order to demonstrate the predictive capabilities of the model	(i) Limitations: (1) The functions α and β could not be determined. Therefore, they were set to be equal to those previously determined for collagen fiber bundles extracted from rat tail tendons. (2) Mechanical response of ligaments is dependent on the strain rate, and thus, experimental data that capture the instantaneous elastic response of the MCLs could be quite different than the quasi-static ones used to determine the constants. (3) Assumption that the deformations of the MCLs are homogeneous.

Table C.2.   (*Continued*)

Study	Country	Setting/context	Participant characteristics	Groups	Outcomes measured
Frigo, CA and Donno, L (2021)	Italy	A musculoskeletal model was developed to analyze the tensions of the knee-joint ligaments during walking and to understand how they change with changes in the muscle forces	Caucasian male (age: 42 years, body height: 1.72 m, body mass: 70 kg)	Model to analyze ligament tensions during walking and to understand how they are affected by muscle contractions	Few studies deal with natural walking, and the results are still questionable. Their musculoskeletal model study provides a contribution to understanding the role of the different muscles in determining the ligaments' loads. (iii) Although the method would require further validation, the main consolidated phenomena about the knee-joint mechanism, like the screw home mechanism, the posterior displacement of the femur during flexion, and the loading/unloading effects on the cruciate ligaments produced by the contraction of quadriceps and hamstrings, were confirmed in their simulations. (iv) Hence, the model appears to be an effective tool for further investigating the biomechanics of knee joint under dynamic conditions.
Shin, CS, Chaudhari, AM and Andriacchi, TP (2007)	USA	Develop, test, and apply a 3D specimen-specific dynamic simulation model of the knee designed to evaluate the influence of deceleration forces during running to a stop (single-leg landing) on ACL strain	The 3D specimen specific knee model	Simulation model was then used to test the balance between ACL strain produced by quadriceps contraction and the reductions in ACL strain associated with the posterior braking force	(i) Assumptions for the model included ligament material properties obtained from the literature rather than the specific material properties of the cadaver specimen. (ii) Model does not account for wrapping of the ACL around the intercondylar notch of the femur or the interaction between the bundles. (iii) ACL strain prediction of the model was validated with a specimen-specific simulation.

Table C.2. (*Continued*)

Study	Country	Setting/context	Participant characteristics	Groups	Outcomes measured
Akalan, NE, Ozkan, M and Temelli, Y (2008)	Turkey?	(i) The purpose of this study is to investigate the effects of anterior portion of anterior cruciate ligament, posterior cruciate ligament, anterior and deep portions of medial collateral ligament, and the tibiofemoral articular contacts on passive knee motion. (ii) Construct a knee model considering the ligament bundles and contact surfaces	NA	Model considering ligament bundles and contact surfaces	They could illustrate that the proposed knee model resembles not only the well- accepted knee models, but also the anatomical findings based on cadaver studies. With this study they intend to get one step closer to understanding the effects of surgical alterations in a virtual environment, by actually modifying anatomically meaningful parameters, such as the lengths of the ligaments, extension or removal of bony tissue.
Bertozzi, L, Stagni, R, Fantozzi, S and Cappello, A (2007)	Italy	Focused on the evaluation of sensitivity of the devised knee model with respect to the cross-sectional area parameter during the A/P translation of the tibia	One living subject	Sensitivity of the model to the cross-sectional area was evaluated during the anterior/posterior tibial translations, and the sensitivity to all the cruciate ligament parameters was evaluated during the internal/external rotations	(i) Each ligament was modeled taking the anatomical twist of the fibers into account. (ii) Sensitivity of the model to the cross-sectional area was evaluated during the anterior/posterior translations of the tibia, and the sensitivity to the cross- sectional area, the reference length, and the elastic modulus was evaluated during the internal/external tibial rotations. (iii) Anterior and the posterior stiffnesses were not very sensitive to variations of the reference length parameter. (iv) Laxity parameter was less influenced than the anterior and the posterior stiffnesses. (v) Good results were obtained with respect to the experimental data. This model featured a good level of accuracy in combination with a very low complexity.

(Continued)

Table C.2.   (*Continued*)

Study	Country	Setting/context	Participant characteristics	Groups	Outcomes measured
Barrett, JM and Callaghan, JP (2017)	Canada	To test whether a mechanistic model of ligamentous tissue portrays behavior representative of the actual ligament failure tests	NA	Model was fitted to experimental average curves for the cervical anterior longitudinal ligament. In addition, the model was cyclically loaded to test whether the tissue model behaves similarly	(i) Key findings that relate to the scoping review question(s). (ii) Model predicts diminished force-producing capacity with repeated submaximal loads, which is consistent with the experimental results. (iii) Model predicts a considerable amount of hysteresis which is also consistent with experimental data: (1) This phenomenon has previously been associated with ligament viscoelasticity. (iv) A natural application of this plastic ligament model would be in characterizing the risk of injury from cumulative loading. (v) Limitations: (1) Viscoelasticity is currently absent from this model. (2) One-dimensional in nature. (3) No input from experiment on the fiber level. (4) Assumed each collagen fiber generates force independently. (5) Each fiber produces force linearly.
Xu, H, Bloswick, D and Merryweather, A (2015)	China	The aim of this study was to develop an OpenSim gait model with enhanced knee structures	NA	Knee rotation affects on the ligaments	(i) Zero-load length is a key parameter used to determine the status of the ligament bundle (recruited or slack): (1) Not directly known and for this study had to be indirectly calculated from reference length and strain. (ii) Length of each ligament bundle is considered as a straight line and is calculated between the femoral and tibial attachment sites in this model: (1) Real ligaments attach over a finite area of the bone and wrap around the bones.

Table C.3.   Characteristics of included studies: Interpretive and critical research form.

Study	Methods for data collection and analysis	Country	Phenomena of interest	Setting/context/ culture	Participant characteristics and sample size	Description of main results
Weiss, JA, Gardiner, JC, Ellis, BJ, Lujan, TJ and Phatak, NS (2005)	(i) Strategies for representing ligaments in joint models: (1) Method 1: A model of the entire joint is constructed including all supporting soft tissue structures: (a) This approach can predict joint kinematics, ligament stresses, strains, insertion site forces, and load transfer to the bones via contact. (b) However, the sheer complexity of these types of models makes this method difficult to implement and the resulting models are nearly impossible to validate without detailed experimental studies. (2) Method 2: A single ligament is represented in the model: (a) This method provides predictions of ligament stress, strains, insertion site forces, and load transfer to the bones via contact, but not kinematics because the motion of the bones to which the ligament is attached must be applied. (ii) Ligament geometry for computational models: (1) Laser scanning and medical imaging are the primary techniques that are used for accurate geometry of the ligaments: (a) Laser scanning: Can be very accurate, but cannot differentiate between the ligament of interest and surrounding bone and soft tissue structures. (b) Medical imaging: 1. Magnetic resonance imaging: Standard MRI pulse sequences do not result in images that have a substantial signal for ligaments, but rather the ligaments structure is shown by a lack of this signal. 2. Computed tomography: CT yields better spatial resolution and a better signal-to-noise ratio, in addition to providing excellent images of the bones around the joint which tend to be important for finite element ligament models.	USA	To describe the strategies for addressing the technical aspects of the computational modeling of ligaments with the finite element method	To describe the strategies for addressing the technical aspects of the computational modeling of ligaments with the finite element method	Literature before 2004	(i) Ligaments can be represented in finite element models using several different strategies. (ii) The choice for geometrical arrangement is dependent on the type of model that is aimed to be created: (1) Can use either laser scanning or medical imaging (MRI or CT) to create the geometry. (iii) Constitutive models are used to describe the behavior of the material of the geometry. (iv) No FE model of a ligament can be fully verified or validated.

(Continued)

Table C.3.   (*Continued*)

Study	Methods for data collection and analysis	Country	Phenomena of interest	Setting/context/ culture	Participant characteristics and sample size	Description of main results
	(iii) Constitutive modeling of ligaments: (1) Constitutive equations are used to describe the mechanical behavior of ideal materials through specification of the dependence of stress on variables such as deformation gradient, rate of deformation, temperature, and pressure. (2) However, the accurate description and prediction of the three-dimensional mechanical behavior of ligaments by constitutive equations remains one of the challenges for computational modeling: (a) This is because the development and application of these models relies on an understanding of ligament structure and function, and a knowledge of available experimental data. (iv) *In-situ* strain: (1) *In-situ* strain is the strain distribution that corresponds to the tension that occurs when a ligament is separated from one of both of its insertions to the bone. (2) Failure to include *in-situ* strain in FE models of ligaments can lead to large errors in the calculations of stress and insertion site forces. (v) Verification and validation: (1) Verification is the process of determining whether or not an FE model of a ligament can be used to represent the underlying principles of continuum mechanics with sufficient accuracy: (a) Verification part 1: Testing the ability of the constitutive models, element technology, contact algorithms, etc. in an FE program to reproduce known analytical solutions to idealized problems with some well-defined error tolerance. (b) Verification part 2: *A-posteriori* error estimation, such as mesh convergence studies. (2) Validation is the comparison of FE model predictions with experimental measurements: (a) There is no way to completely verify or validate an FE model of ligament mechanics					

Table C.4.   Characteristics of included studies: Analytical cross-sectional study form.

Study	Country	Setting/context	Participant characteristics	Groups	Outcomes measured
Barrett, JM and Callaghan, JP (2018)	Ontario, Canada	To present a straightforward three-step method for determining three model parameters (k: the ligaments' effective stiffness; μ: the average collagen slack length; and σ: standard deviation of collagen slack lengths) of ligaments from the force–deflection data	Force–deflection data from Mattucci (2011) for anterior longitudinal ligament of the middle cervical spine (C4–C6) of males loaded at a low strain rate	Compared their step-wise procedure results to those obtained from a nonlinear least-square method fitted to the same experimental data	Ligament force–displacement parameters in the toe and linear regions can be analytically derived using this three-step method. Although these parameters have yet to be quantified, the study highlights their interaction with the force–elongation curve of ligaments.
Nasseri, A, Khataee, H, Bryant, AL and Lloyd, DG (2020)	Australia	To develop and validate a computational model that predicts the force applied to the ACL in response to knee loading in three planes of motion	Experimental data from female participants during a dynamic task	Validated computational model by comparing results to the cadaveric experimental data that predicted ACL force	A validated computational model can successfully analyze ligaments.
Provenzano, P, Lakes, R, Keenan, T and vanderby Jr., R (2001)	Wisconsin, USA	In this study, two viscoelastic properties are considered: The increase in tissue deformation over time with a constant load (creep) and the decrease in load with time at a constant tissue elongation (stress relaxation). The authors' hypothesis is that nonlinear viscoelasticity of ligament requires a description more general than the separable QLV formulation commonly used. To test this hypothesis, both creep and relaxation experiments were performed at multiple levels in the physiologic region of recoverable loading	Eighteen medial collateral ligaments from euthanized Sprague–Dawley male rats were used	Creep and relaxation studies at various loads and deformations below the damage threshold	(i) Results show a nonlinear behavior in which the rate of creep is dependent on the stress level and the rate of relaxation is dependent on the strain level. (ii) Relaxation occurs faster than creep. (iii) These results are not consistent with the quasi-linear viscoelastic theory of behavior for ligaments.

(Continued)

Table C.4.   (*Continued*)

Study	Country	Setting/context	Participant characteristics	Groups	Outcomes measured
Ozada, N (2015)	Turkey	The study's objective was to model the contributions of the collateral ligaments over six degrees of freedom (DOFs) of knee-joint articulation to aid the diagnosis of knee-ligament injuries	The 3D image scan of knee	Two sets of calculations were made: (1) six-DOF kinematics of the knee, and (2) changes in MCL and LCL lengths. Results were obtained under three different conditions: (1) the intact knee with all major ligaments and cartilage attached; (2) the MCL completely removed; and (3) the LCL completely removed. The three-DOF translations (anterior–posterior, medial–lateral, and superior–inferior) and two-DOF rotations (varus–valgus and internal–external) were presented from one-DOF tibial flexion–extension	(i) A combined focus from clinicians and researchers on joint modeling and the use of modeling-based results in clinical practice may help to predict joint behavior after treatment that may be difficult to observe empirically and is generalizable to different types of joint replacements. (ii) Describes six-DOF kinematics of the tibia with MCL or LCL removed and establishes the general reference axis of bodies such as the center of mass. (iii) These findings may be useful for the knee arthroplasty research of collateral ligament injuries and for developing approaches to restore ligament tension in six DOFs.
Yang, Z, Wickwire, AC and Debski, RE (2010)	Pennsylvania, USA	The objective of this study was to develop a subject-specific model of the knee that is kinematically driven to predict the forces in the major ligaments at high flexion angles	One freshly thawed 25-year-old male cadaveric knee	(i) The forces in the ACL, PCL, MCL, and LCL were determined using the testing system in position control mode for use in the optimization procedure. (ii) The experimental load–elongation curves representing the PCL, MCL, and LCL were then fit to fourth-order polynomials	(i) This study developed a kinematically driven, subject-specific model of a cadaveric knee for high flexion angles based on geometry obtained from an MR dataset; kinematic and ligament force data in response to external loading conditions; and load–elongation curves from structural tests of each ligament. (ii) The predictions from the model were compared with the experimental data and the optimization criterion was satisfied since 92% of the comparisons met the optimization criterion that was based on the repeatability of the robotic/UFS testing system.

Table C.4.   (*Continued*)

Study	Country	Setting/context	Participant characteristics	Groups	Outcomes measured
Beidokhti, HN, Janssen, D, van de Groes, S, Hazrati, J, Van den Boogaard, T and Verdonschot, N (2017)	Australia	The aim of this study was to evaluate the effects of: (1) the ligament modeling approach [nonlinear springs (1D) versus transversely isotropic continuum (3D) models]; and (2) the selection of the data used to describe the behavior of ligaments (based on either the literature or subject-specific optimization)	Three fresh-frozen cadavers with no signs of injuries or surgery	The effect of modeling choices on the predictive capability of FE models of the human knee joint	(i) When modeling the knee joint in FE, adopting subject-specific material parameters affects and improves the quality of the model Predictions. (ii) Comparing with the ligament spring representations used in this study, using a continuum modeling approach results in more accurate contact outcome variables: (1) However, when mainly the prediction of joint kinematics is of interest, the spring ligament Models provide a faster option. (iii) In high flexion, representing the ligaments with multiple spring elements covering the ligament insertion sites is recommended. (iv) The method implemented in this study can be adapted to *in-vivo* patient-specific FE modeling to assess the biomechanical behavior of the joint, as all the main tibiofemoral ligament material properties were calculated based on the tests which can be performed noninvasively.
Innocenti, B, Salandra, P, Pascale, W and Pianigiani, S (2016)	Amsterdam, the Netherlands	This study aimed to define and validate a method for the accuracy and reproducibility of MRI scans in identifying cruciate and collateral ligament insertions	Left and right knee MRI scans from Mimics 17.0	Two groups of three operators with different medical imaging processing experiences independently applied the procedure on MRI scans for a total of 10 fresh-frozen full-leg cadavers with nonarthritic knees	(i) The results showed that the procedure was not only reproducible but also accurate with possible general variability of < 1 mm, with the exception of collateral ligaments, for which an error of 3 mm could be expected: (1) This average result could be considered acceptable under the assumption that the insertion areas of collateral ligaments are identified by only one point, as the barycenter, and that this point cannot be precisely recognized, especially for large insertion areas such as the MCL. (ii) Analysis of lower-image-quality scans still gave acceptable results, although these were inferior to those for the MRIs with medium–high image quality. (iii) Limitations: (1) Localization defined using only points: (a) Defining the real area could be useful for several clinical and biomechanical aspects. (2) This study was performed using only healthy knees: (a) Knees with pathological conditions could be studied as well.

(*Continued*)

Table C.4.   (*Continued*)

Study	Country	Setting/context	Participant characteristics	Groups	Outcomes measured
Mommersteeg, TJA, Huiskes, R, Blankevoort, L, Kooloos, JGM, Kauer, JMG and Maathuis, PGM (1997)	The Netherlands	This study aimed to assess the resultant force vectors and force distributions in all human knee ligaments simultaneously by using a new method comprised of the inverse dynamics modeling approach	One freshly frozen cadaveric knee joint that didn't have any signs of knee pathology	(1) Determining the joint motions associated with externally applied anterior–posterior forces. (2) Determining the relationships between ligament forces and the relative positions of the bones. (3) Determining the insertion site geometry of bundles identified in the ligaments. (4) Determining the bundle force–length relationships by combining steps (2) and (3). (5) Determining the forces in the bundles by combining the steps (1), (3), and (4).	(i) Using an inverse dynamics approach provides a feasible method for obtaining detailed 3D load distributions of knee ligament simultaneously. (ii) The forces in several bundles of more than one ligament can be determined simultaneously. (iii) The way in which the parameters describing force–length relationships of the ligament bundles are identified conquers two problems common in ligament testing: (1) Ligament properties have been shown to depend on the alignment of the ligament in the testing machine: (a) Using this study's method, the test orientations are varied and the variable ligament behavior is accounted for in the analysis. (2) This method offers a solution for the problem of the zero-load length determination of the ligament bundles. (iv) The multi-line representations of the ligaments are based on actual measurements of the anatomy: (1) In the past, ligaments have been modeled using two or three arbitrary line elements based on the measurements of the ligament insertion site parameters: (a) Using two or three line elements has been shown to not stabilize the knee during its entire range of motion. (v) Advantages to this method: (1) No external devices must be attached to the ligaments: (a) These external devices can cause impingement problems or alterations in the load–elongation behavior of the ligament. (2) The joint remains intact during the kinematic experiment which preserves the anatomic relationships within the joint: (a) In dissection studies, the removal of a supporting structure might influence the internal configuration of remaining knee-joint

Table C.4.   (*Continued*)

Study	Country	Setting/context	Participant characteristics	Groups	Outcomes measured
					structures, altering their role in knee-joint mechanics. (b) The ligaments provide direct restraints caused by interaction between ligaments and their articular surfaces. (3) This method is not limited with respect to the complexity of the knee loading configuration and the DOFs of the test. (vi) Limitations to this method: (1) Method is time-consuming and technologically involved. (2) Ligaments are represented by a number of line elements which do not interact with each other: (a) The effects of mechanical bundle-matrix and inter-bundle interactions were assumed to be neglected. (3) The ACL was shown using longitudinal separation of the anterior and posterior portions of the ligament which minimally influence the stiffness of the knee in anterior tibial loading: (a) This could be a factor that affects the accuracy of this method. (4) It was assumed that the multi-line-element models can extrapolate information to other ligament orientations which occur *in-situ*, but these were not represented in the bench tests
Jiang, Y, Wang, Y and Peng, X (2015)	Shanghai, China	To develop a constitutive model for human ligaments that is visco-hyperelastic fiber-reinforced and contains an energy density function that is decomposed into two parts	Experimental data of strain rate-dependent properties of younger human cervical spine ligaments was used	Compared the material parameters derived with experimental data	The results indicate that the model presented here can properly characterize the visco-hyperelastic biomechanical behavior of human spine ligaments.

(*Continued*)

Table C.4.   (*Continued*)

Study	Country	Setting/context	Participant characteristics	Groups	Outcomes measured
Akbar, M, Farahmand, F and Arjmand, N (2019)	Amsterdam, the Netherlands	(i) The purpose of this study was to propose a methodology for mechanical characterization of the ligaments in subject-specific models of the patellofemoral joint (PFJ) of living individuals. (ii) It was hypothesized that characterization of the mechanical properties of the ligaments in a geometrically subject-specific PFJ model could improve the model's predictions for the joint stability behavior, as required for surgical preplanning applications	Healthy male volunteer (180 cm, 84 kg and 30 years), with no history of PFJ disorder, participated in this study	Sensitivity analyses were performed to investigate the effect of mechanical properties of the noncharacterized model components on the characterization procedure and its results	(i) This study is a first step toward truly subject-specific modeling of the PFJ of living individuals, to be used for personalized preplanning of the clinical interventions in patients suffering from joint disorders. (ii) To the best of their knowledge, this study is the first in the literature that utilizes *in-vivo* characterization tests for subject-specific modeling of the PFJ, although a similar approach has been employed previously for modeling of the cadaver joints using *in-vitro* experiments. (iii) Limitations: (1) Only included the MPFL, the LPFL, and the patellar tendon, as the joint's passive structures, neglecting the effects associated with other soft tissues, such as patellotibial and patellominiscal ligaments, retinacula, and joint capsule. (2) MPFL and LPFL were modeled as nonlinear elastic materials and their viscoelastic behavior was neglected. (3) Mechanical properties of the noncharacterized model components, i.e. the stiffnesses of the articular cartilage and the patellar tendon, and the specific strain stiffness constant and the pre-strain of the quadriceps muscles were based on the literature and were not subject-specific.

Table C.4. (*Continued*)

Study	Country	Setting/context	Participant characteristics	Groups	Outcomes measured
Alzakerin, HM, Halkiadakis, Y and Morgan, KD (2021)	USA	This study sought to employ computational modeling to investigate differences in how the ACL is loaded during running in healthy controls and post-ACLR individuals	Sixteen post-ACLR and 12 healthy controls performed a running protocol	Sixteen post- ACLR individuals (age: 19.5 ± 6.3 years; mass: 70.1 ± 11 kg; height: 1.7 ± 0.1 m, speed: 2.7 ± 0.3 m/s; and gender: eight males and eight females), 12 healthy controls (age: 21.2 ± 4.3 years; mass: 63.3 ± 14.6 kg; height: 1.7 ± 0.1 m, speed: 2.6 ± 0.3 m/s; and gender: six males and six females)	Force in the ACL was computed as a function of the change in ACL length and the linear elastic stiffness of ACL.
Hui, C, Pi, Y, Swami, V, Mabee, M and Jaremko, JL (2016)	Canada	To test the validity of the ACL insertion sites identified using their 3D modeling program and to determine the accuracy of arthroscopic ACL reconstruction guided by their "virtual arthroscopic" model	Sixteen cadaveric knees	Mean lengths of the anteromedial and posterolateral bundles in the sagittal plane and width of the anteromedial and posterolateral bundles in the sagittal and coronal planes were calculated automatically by their program for each examiner and for both examiners combined	(i) Developed a novel tool using routine knee MRI sequences that can identify the centers of the ACL femoral and tibial footprints accurately and reliably, thereby allowing for the creation of a 3D model that can be digitally rotated into a "virtual arthroscopic" view, simulating the arthroscopic views observed in the operating Room. (ii) Key concern with anatomic single-bundle ACL reconstruction is that the ideal tunnel position has not yet been established. (iii) Sample size, although substantial for a cadaveric study and justified by power analysis, was still small. (iv) Surgeon bias in the two specimens with significant anatomic variability to the ACL femoral footprint visualized on MRI.

(Continued)

Table C.4.   (*Continued*)

Study	Country	Setting/context	Participant characteristics	Groups	Outcomes measured
Sun, C, Miao, F, Wang, X-M, Wang, T, Ma, R, Wang, D-P and Liu, C (2008)	China	To study the clinical application of dual-energy CT in the knee ligaments	Twenty-four knees scanned	(i) Data obtained from DECT were transferred to a workstation (Volume Wizard) and images of the knee were reconstructed by multi-planar reconstruction (MPR) and volume rendering technique (VRT). (ii) Rotated to different positions in order to observe the 3D and multi-location images of the knee	(i) Differentiation of collagen makes it possible to depict ligaments and ligaments could also be multi-angled and displayed three-dimensionally. (ii) MRI is the golden standard for examining intra-articular structures of the knee and surrounding soft tissue (Adeeb *et al.*, 2004), but no reports had been found on the fact that MRI could display the tendon and ligament in three dimensions, since the spatial resolution of MR scans is not achieved. (iii) DECT could also give a multi-angled image of the tendon and ligament. (iv) Limitations of DECT: (1) Thinner and transverse ligaments, such as the tibial collateral ligament, the lateral patellar retinaculum, and medial patellar retinaculum, were displayed not so satisfactorily. (2) Because of the coverage of its rear muscles, the posterior ligament, such as oblique popliteal ligament, could not be shown clearly. (3) Scanning time that DECT used for the knee is about two–three times of MSCT.

Table C.4.   (*Continued*)

Study	Country	Setting/context	Participant characteristics	Groups	Outcomes measured
Tan, J, Mu, M, Liao, G, Zhao, Y and Li, J (2015)	China	This study biomechanically explored the pathological changes during Monteggia fractures using finite element analysis	Two cadaveric forearm specimens underwent computed tomography in both the prone and supine positions	The mechanical changes of the annular ligament in the two positions were observed and compared.	(i) Limitations: (1) FEA cannot perfectly simulate the real situation that occurs during injury due to the complexity of human anatomic structures and the imperfections of the FEA software. (2) With the development of computer-aided engineering software, this shortcoming of FEA may be overcome. (3) It is difficult to obtain sufficient fresh specimens (without preservative): (a) The properties of the intersection of the annular ligament and capsule could be greatly affected by preservatives. (b) Although the mechanical property values were assigned to the bone and the ligament according to the literature, the final property values could be affected by the thickness of the cortical and cancellous bones in different specimens. (c) It would be theoretically better to increase the number of specimens to obtain mean values for the structural indices.

(*Continued*)

Table C.4.   (*Continued*)

Study	Country	Setting/context	Participant characteristics	Groups	Outcomes measured
Tuna, M, Sunbuloglu, E and Bozdag, E (2014)	Kidlington, UK	The aim of this study is to formulate a user-specified contact model that can be used in conjunction with finite element software and reflects PDL's influence on the neighboring structures based on the currently available information, without requiring an actual volumetric finite element mesh of ligament	One randomly selected patient	(i) Aim of this study is to formulate a user-specified contact model that can be used in conjunction with finite element software and reflects PDL's influence on the neighboring structures based on the currently available information, without requiring an actual volumetric finite element mesh of ligament	(i) In dental biomechanics, the inclusion of periodontal ligament into FE studies is essential. However, including it as a 3D mesh yields an increase in the total element number, preprocessing and computational times, along with indispensable memory requirements. (ii) The proposed model mimics PDL behavior via a custom contact algorithm, transmits stress among the tooth and the alveolar bone but does not require a physical 3D mesh of the ligament.
Mommersteeg, TJ, Blankevoort, L, Huiskes, R, Kooloos, JG and Kauer, JM (1996)	The Netherlands	During knee-joint motions, the fiber bundles of the knee ligaments are nonuniformly loaded in a recruitment pattern, which depends on successive relative orientations of the insertion sites. These fiber bundles vary with respect to length, orientation, and mechanical properties. As a result, the stiffness characteristics of the ligaments as a whole are variable during knee-joint motion. The purpose of this study is to characterize this variable mechanical behavior	Six ligaments from three human knee joints	Subfailure ligament tests performed in different relative insertion orientations, were simulated	(i) The hypothesis that a multi-bundle concept is essential to characterize fully the mechanical behavior of human knee ligaments, is verified. (ii) More detailed specimen-based line element representations of the ligaments were obtained of which the nonuniform stiffness and recruitment parameters were also determined. (iii) As in all studies in which a mathematical model is applied to experimental observations, the model parameters can be estimated only adequately from the experiment if the number of observations is attuned to the number of parameters.

Table C.4.   (*Continued*)

Study	Country	Setting/context	Participant characteristics	Groups	Outcomes measured
Kernozek, TW and Ragan, RJ (2008)	USA	A phenomenological sagittal plane model was used to estimate the ACL tension during drop-landing from the net knee moments and forces, obtained from inverse dynamics and electromyography	Sixteen female athletes [mean age = 22 years (range 20–23), mean height = 170.2 (SD = 5.38) cm, and mean weight = 62.6 (SD = 6.2) kg]	ACL tension during drop-landing from the net knee moments and forces	(i) Limitations: (1) Error is introduced by inaccuracies in placing markers relative to bony landmarks, the amount of skin, muscle, and other soft tissue movements related to skeletal motion. (2) Participant and cadaveric age were not similar, potentially influencing numerous parameters used. (3) Moment exerted by the gastrocnemius in the model was not straightforward to calculate due to the two-joint nature of this muscle group. (4) Quasi-static ligament behavior used in this investigation may not describe the ligament behavior under rapid, dynamic loads.
Luetkemeyer, CM, Scheven, U, Estrada, JB and Arruda, EM (2021)	USA	This work demonstrates that (when strain heterogeneity and structural properties are accounted for) ligament material properties are deterministic and ligament material microstructure is detectable with mesoscale measures of mechanical function	Five ovine tibiofemoral Joints	Explaining their entire material characterization process step-by-step, from experimental measurements to computational inverse modeling, beginning with an overview of each piece of information that is required for the VFM-based inverse algorithm (see Sec. 2.1). The material modeling methods presented here account for full-volume heterogeneous deformation (measured with displacement-encoded MRI, as described in Sec. 2.3), heterogeneous material direction (fiber splay, as described in Sec. 2.5), and curved, 3D displacement boundary conditions (enthesis shapes, as described in Sec. 2.6)	(i) While most of the constitutive parameters found were consistent between groups, significantly larger values of κ were found for the PL bundles of the ACL compared to both AM bundles and PTs when the HGO model was used: (1) This difference indicates a higher degree of collagen fiber alignment in AM bundles and PTs compared to PL bundles. Smaller values for κ in the HGO-MAC model and smaller values of a or larger values of b in the tFJC model also suggest that the AM bundle and PT have a higher degree of anisotropy (i.e. collagen alignment) than the PL bundle, although the differences were not significant. (ii) This study, however, is the first to detect this microstructural difference with mechanical measurements alone. (iii) Limitations: (1) The virtual displacement fields (or test functions) used were user-defined, chosen to be reasonable and subject to the boundary conditions: (a) When different virtual fields were used, slightly different material

(*Continued*)

Table C.4.   (*Continued*)

Study	Country	Setting/context	Participant characteristics	Groups	Outcomes measured
					parameter estimates were obtained, but the same trends were observed. Recent works have introduced ideas for automating and optimizing the construction of virtual fields. (2) Experimental measurement noise can cause parameter estimates to be less precise and less accurate. (3) It remains unclear what material model form is most suitable for ligaments, let alone how to estimate the accuracy of identified parameters. (4) It is also likely that the simple experimental test used (unidirectional tension) did not create enough variability in the deformation gradient tensor field to provide the inverse method with the information necessary to correctly identify all material parameters for all specimens. (5) Construction of the full-volume fiber direction fields could also be improved: (a) Local material direction was estimated based on linear interpolations from each specimen's outer edges. (6) It is likely that more data may have revealed more significant differences between groups. (7) This study considered material nonlinearity and anisotropy. However, ligaments are also viscoelastic, meaning their response is time/history-dependent.

Table C.4.   (*Continued*)

Study	Country	Setting/context	Participant characteristics	Groups	Outcomes measured
Kar, J and Quesada, PM (2013)	USA	It demonstrates a technique for estimating the dynamic changes to knee and ACL variables by conducting musculoskeletal simulation on motion analysis data, collected from actual stop-jump tasks performed by young recreational women athletes	Eleven young recreational female athletes, with average body weight of 59.7 ± 7.7 (1 SD) kg, height of 164.4 ± 12.7 cm, and median age of 20 years, were classified as recreational athletes since they participated in group or individual athletic activities on a regular basis	ACL strain and internal force developed during real-time stop-jump activities	(i) Limitations: (1) Restricting knee sagittal plane translations as functions of flexion only: (a) Tibiofemoral translation in the vertical direction is interrelated with valgus where valgus-induced tibiofemoral separation would increase ACL strain and internal force. (2) Not using internal–external rotational DOF and it possibly restricted the knee transverse plane translation, particularly in the anterior–posterior direction perpendicular to the frontal plane: (a) IE rotation, particularly occurring in the mid-flexion range, 30–60°, which tries to cause larger tibiofemoral separation in the anterior–posterior direction, is primarily opposed by the ACL. (b) A shorter anterior–posterior separation would result in less strains and internal forces at the ACL. (c) For better accuracy the IE rotational DOF needs to be unconstrained and the knee anterior–posterior translational DOF to be made a function of both flexion and IE rotational DOF. (3) Lack of modeling important biomechanical elements that contribute to knee-joint motion and orientation, mainly three other knee ligaments. (4) Representing ACL as a single bundle of fibers (not with separate AM and PL bundles) can be considered a limitation, given the current trends in practicing double-bundle ACL reconstruction surgeries. (5) Study population of female-only subjects.

(*Continued*)

Table C.4.   (*Continued*)

Study	Country	Setting/context	Participant characteristics	Groups	Outcomes measured
Haraguchi, N, Armiger, RS, Myerson, MS, Campbell, JT and Chao, EYS (2009)	USA	The goal was to quantify and visualize the three-dimensional loading relationship between the ligaments and articular surfaces of the ankle to identify and determine the stabilizing roles of these anatomical structures during the stance phase of gait	Five subjects	Analyzed joint contact pressures and periankle ligament tension concurrently	(i) Limitations: (1) Loading conditions were calculated only for positions in the sagittal plane. (2) Far more tendons crossing the ankle than were considered in this study. (3) Stiffness properties of the joint cartilage and some of the ligaments are not currently available and had to be extrapolated. (4) Model did not have complete freedom of motion of any bone except the fibula and was thus over-constrained. (5) Because they assumed that the fibula was rigid, force in the distal tibiofibular ligaments and the interosseous membrane might have been overestimated. (6) Specific experimental testing with cadaveric specimens is needed to validate their results.
Adouni, M, Mbarki, R, Al Khatib, F and Eilaghi, A (2021)	Australia	To develop a multi-scale constitutive model that considers the structural hierarchies of soft tissues	Forty-six control samples of knee ligament/tendons from human donors collected during uniaxial tensile tests	Model creates a relationship between the aggregate mechanical behavior of the soft tissues and the basic microscale properties predicted by molecular dynamics simulations	Model predictions are in agreement with the results of experimental and numerical studies. Proposed model is of clinical significance as it facilitates the understanding of hormone-mediated changes to the full joint mechanics and provides insights into the etiology of gender bias. (iii) Limitations: (1) Full elastoplastic matrix was not used. (2) Three different sets of experimental data were used during the calibration of the model. (3) Model sensitivity to the geometry aspect was not considered. (4) Full model calibration, starting from molecular measurement/prediction to macromechanical behavior of the connective tissue, was not considered. (5) Current results and conclusions remain limited to the short-term ligament response.

Table C.4.   (*Continued*)

Study	Country	Setting/context	Participant characteristics	Groups	Outcomes measured
Seth, A, Sherman, M, Reinbolt, JA and Delp, SL (2011)	USA	(i) Providing overview of OpenSim. (ii) To discuss a model developed to study walking and applied to gain deeper insights into muscle and focus on the aims of *in-vivo* experiments with a postural stability platform and a human model that provide a research environment for performing human posture experiments *in-silico*	NA	Overview of OpenSim	(i) Model ligaments that compute force as a function of positions and velocities from the state. (ii) Tension generated by ligament is dependent only on path length and velocity.
Wren, TAL, Beaupre, GS and Carter, DR (1997)	USA	To develop an analytical framework for quantitatively describing changes in uniaxial tendon and ligament properties throughout ontogeny. In this approach, cross-sectional area, modulus, and strength undergo baseline levels of development due to inherent time-dependent biological influences	(i) Different animals: (1) rabbit Achilles tendon and (2) rat tail tendon	Relationships linking changes in tendon and ligament properties to biological influences and mechanical loading	(i) To their knowledge, this is the first attempt at applying analytical methods to study tendon and ligament growth, development, and adaptation in the context of experimental findings. (ii) This model provides insight into tendon and ligament adaptation beyond that provided by experimental studies. (iii) They have proposed basic principles that help to explain the growth and development of tendons and ligaments: (1) These principles appear to apply not only to normal growth and development, but also to growth and development under conditions of increased or decreased loading.

(*Continued*)

Table C.4.   *(Continued)*

Study	Country	Setting/context	Participant characteristics	Groups	Outcomes measured
Gasparutto, X, Sancisi, N, Jacquelin, E, Parenti-Castelli, V and Dumas, R (2015)	France, Italy	The objective of this study was to validate, against *in-vivo* knee-joint kinematics measured by intra-cortical pins on three subjects, the model-based kinematics obtained by MBO methods using three different types of ligament constraints	Three subjects	MBO methods validated against *in-vivo* knee-joint angles and displacements	(i) Study presented encouraging results for the use of anatomical constraints in MBO. (ii) Limitations: (1) Running cycles were acquired with only three cameras and the data suffered from occlusions. (2) Knee geometry on which the anatomical constraints introduced in the MBO depend was not personalized in this study, and can only represent a nonpathological knee.
Bertozzi, L, Stagni, R, Fantozzi, S and Cappello, A (2008)	Italy	The objective of this study was to evaluate a cruciate ligament model that could achieve this knowledge while avoiding any destructive measurements in living healthy subjects	A living subject	Laxity, anterior, and posterior stiffnesses were calculated and compared with the literature	(i) Laxity was most sensitive to reference length but fitted the literature well considering the reference length estimated from the subject. (ii) Both stiffnesses were most sensitive to elastic modulus variations. (iii) At full extension, anterior stiffness overestimated the literature, but at 90° good comparisons with the literature were obtained. (iv) Posterior stiffness showed smaller overestimations. (v) Devised model, when properly improved, could evaluate the role of the cruciate ligaments of a living subject during the execution of daily living activities.

Table C.4.   (*Continued*)

Study	Country	Setting/context	Participant characteristics	Groups	Outcomes measured
Forestiero, A, Carniel, EL, Fontanella, CG and Natali, AN (2017)	Australia	This study's aim is to provide a computational tool for the investigation of ankle mechanics under different loading conditions, and in specific, the biomechanical role of ankle ligaments	CT imaging for bones, MRI imaging for soft tissue and skin of a 58-year-old male	Healthy ankle versus injured ankle	(i) This study's procedure provides a computational tool for the investigation of the biomechanics of healthy and injured hindfoot ligaments: (1) The results allow one to identify the mechanical response of the foot in healthy conditions, and the mechanical response of the ligaments during ankle movements. (ii) This computational tool allows the investigation of the foot response in the case of ankle joint trauma (i.e. severe sprains or ruptures). (iii) Limitations of this method: (1) The exclusion of specific clinical cases that present some morphologic problems or particular ankle conformation (i.e. claw or flat foot). (2) The reliability of the procedure is evaluated through the comparison between numerical results and experimental data for one subject: (a) Therefore, morphological differences due to the subject variability produce marginal discrepancies between the model and the experimental results.
Seo, Y-J, Yoo, Y-S, Noh, K-C, Song, S-Y, Lee, Y-B, Kim, H-J and Kim, HY (2012)	France	The aim of this study was to determine the acromioclavicular (AC) motion and changes in length and tension of the coracoclavicular ligament during different positions of shoulder abduction using a three-dimensional finite element model based on computed tomography images from normal human shoulders	Right shoulders of 10 living subjects were scanned	Tension and length changes of each ligament during shoulder abduction were assessed	(i) One of the most important findings of this study is that the motion of the AC joint is greater than indicated in previous studies. (ii) Limitations: (1) Assumed that both ligaments were incompressible hyperelastic materials, although actual *in-vivo* ligaments are compressible and viscoelastic: (a) Compared only the patterns of stress distribution at the conoid and trapezoid ligaments and did not seek to determine the absolute values of equivalent stresses. (2) Stress patterns were considered only at discrete abduction angles, rather than as a continuum. (3) Assumed that the outlines of footprints would not be 100% accurate compared with cadaveric models: (a) To decrease error, shoulder models were constructed as precisely as possible to delineate the outlines of each footprint by reproducing marginal ridges, which were considered to be the borderlines of footprints.

(*Continued*)

Table C.4.   (*Continued*)

Study	Country	Setting/context	Participant characteristics	Groups	Outcomes measured
Bolcos, PO, Mononen, ME, Mohammadi, A, Ebrahimi, M, Tanaka, MS, Samaan, MA, Souza, RB, Li, X, Suomalainen, J-S, Toyras, J and Korhonen, RK (2018)	USA, London	In this study, more complex, kinetic-driven (forces and moments) and simpler, kinetic–kinematic-driven (forces and angles) finite element models were compared during the stance phase of gait	One subject	Compare the predictions of kinetic- and kinetic–kinematic-driven knee-joint models in terms of contact mechanics and mechanical response of cartilage during the stance phase of gait	(i) These results suggest that simpler models, in terms of motion and geometry, could be applied when analyzing specific kinetic and kinematic parameters and especially cartilage stresses and strains for large patient cohorts. (ii) Limitations: (1) Only one subject was included in the study. (2) Total joint force was produced primarily by the translational forces and ligament forces, due to their pre-strains and stiffnesses, together with quadriceps forces pulling the patella in the most complex model, similarly as has been done before. (3) Lack of direct experimental validation.
Baldwin, MA, Clary, CW, Fitzpatrick, CK, Deacy, JS, Maletsky, LP and Rullkoetter, PJ (2012)	USA	The purpose of this study was to develop and verify a computational model of a dynamic, whole joint knee simulator	Three fresh-frozen unmatched cadaver left knees	Measure the accuracy of predicted six-DOF TF and PF kinematics during two force-driven, PID-controlled dynamic activities in the KKS	(i) Agreement was demonstrated in trend and magnitude between model-predicted and experimental six-DOF tibiofemoral and patellofemoral kinematics in all three specimen-specific implanted cadaver models during the generation of dynamic, force-driven models of simulated deep knee bend and gait activities in the mechanical Kansas knee simulator. (ii) Limitations: (1) Tuning ligament structures to specimen-specific experimental data can be relatively time-consuming.
Naserkhaki, S, Arjmand, N, Shirazi-Adl, A, Farahmand, F and El-Rich, M (2018)	Iran, Canada, and UAE	This study aims to investigate the relative effects of eight different ligament property datasets on FE model responses	A 20-year-old male	Properties of ligaments versus FE model responses	(i) Large variations in responses were computed with none of the models predicting responses that match all experimental data on RoM, IDP, CoR, ligament force/strain, and moment-sharing. (ii) Using some datasets, however, resulted in closer agreement with the experimental data. (iii) Limitations: (1) Relative performances of various ligament models could also markedly be affected by large inter-subject variations in geometry and remaining material properties. (2) A rigid restraint placed on the superior endplate and facets at the L4 level to displace together during loading could influence strains and forces in ligaments in various models.

Table C.4. (*Continued*)

Study	Country	Setting/context	Participant characteristics	Groups	Outcomes measured
Smale, KB, Conconi, M, Sancisi, N, Krogsgaard, M, Alkjaer, T, Parenti-Castelli, V and Benoit, DL (2019)	Canada	The purpose of this study was to determine if the inclusion of an MRI-based knee model would elicit differences in lower limb kinematics and resulting knee ligament lengths during a side-cut task	Eleven ACL-deficient patients (four females and seven males; 28.3 ± 5.4 years; 175.1 ± 8.5 cm; and 77.2 ± 14.3 kg). Inclusion criteria are primary ACL injury and no history of contralateral ACL ruptures	Lower limb kinematics	(i) MRI-based knee model is responsive to the kinematics and ligament lengths of highly dynamic tasks and may prove to be the most valid option for continuing with late-stage modeling operations such as static optimization. (ii) Limitations: (1) Even though ligament insertion sites on the MRI are identified as point clouds, a single point within these clouds to produce the most isometric fiber of each ligament is used to determine the optimum insertion points and length: (a) It naturally leads to a more conservative estimate in length changes but was a necessary assumption when trying to implement patient-specific parameters into an OpenSim model (needs a more advanced MRI analysis). (2) Relatively small framing of the MRIs: (a) Originally intended for diagnostic purposes and therefore do not include the full femur, tibia, and fibula. (3) Even though considerable differences were observed amongst the four different models, the actual *in-vivo* motions remain unknown. (4) Use of spherical approximations for the two condylar contacts.

(*Continued*)

Table C.4.   (*Continued*)

Study	Country	Setting/context	Participant characteristics	Groups	Outcomes measured
Charles, JP, Fu, FH and Anderst, WJ (2021)	USA	This study demonstrates the sensitivity of ACL force predictions to SS anatomy, specifically musculoskeletal joint geometry and ligament resting lengths, as well as the feasibility for generating SS musculoskeletal models for a group of subjects to predict *in-vivo* tissue loading during functional activities	Ten individuals (five males and five females; age: 27 ± 4 years; and body mass: 76 ± 12 kg).	Passive forces exerted by the ACL during a full cycle of level treadmill walking in uninjured knees	(i) Patterns of ligament forces in both ACL bundles predicted here in the SS models follow the patterns of relative elongation reported by Nagai *et al.* (2019). (ii) These data partially supported Hypothesis 1, although it is possible that small adjustments to the ligament attachment points within the scaled-generic models, particularly those of the ACL, could improve the force predictions of the scaled-generic models and result in closer matches to the subject-specific predictions. (iii) The resting length of these ligaments (the length beyond which they begin to develop a passive force) is another important input factor in these ligament models, but one which is usually estimated rather than directly measured in studies modeling the dynamic behavior of knee ligaments. (iv) Limitations: (1) While a good agreement in predicted ACL forces was seen in the SS models to previous musculoskeletal modeling studies, comparisons such as these do little to assess the true validity of the models or their outputs. (2) Despite the high accuracy of the knee joints in each subject-specific model created here, with high-resolution musculoskeletal geometry, six degrees of joint freedom, and individualized joint centers of rotation based on anatomical landmarks, these centers of rotation were fixed throughout each walking gait cycle. (3) Investigating downhill running, cutting, or pivot maneuvers, which place more load on the ACL, would be more relevant to predictions of postsurgical rehabilitation.

Table C.4. (*Continued*)

Study	Country	Setting/context	Participant characteristics	Groups	Outcomes measured
Weinhandl, JT, Earl-Boehm, JE, Ebersole, KT, Huddleston, WE, Armstrong, BSR and O'Connor, KM (2014)	USA	The purpose of this study was to determine the influence of hamstring strength on anterior cruciate ligament loading during the anticipated sidestep cut	Seventeen recreationally active females [age: 21 (1) years, mass: 61.7 (6.8) kg, and height: 1.66 (0.05) m] participated in this investigation. Participants were physically active [participation in running and cutting activities (i.e. soccer, volleyball, tennis, and basketball) at least 30 min per day, 3 days per week] and had no history of lower extremity or back injury within 6 months prior to the participation or surgery in either lower extremity or the back	Influence of hamstring strength on ACL loading during a sidestep cut	(i) Limitations: (1) CMC was utilized to estimate muscle activations which uses a combination of proportional-derivative control and static optimization. (2) Model parameters such as posterior tibial slope and muscle force line of action were based on average cadaveric data. (3) ACL loads calculated for each plane in this investigation may not be linearly additive under combined loading. (4) Sidestep cutting task utilized in this study was an anticipated task where the participants knew exactly what to expect.
Weinhandl, JT, Earl-Boehm, JE, Ebersole, KT, Huddleston, WE, Armstrong, BSR and O'Connor, KM (2013)	USA	The purpose of this study was to determine the influence of movement anticipation on anterior cruciate ligament loading using a musculoskeletal modeling approach	Twenty healthy recreationally active females [age: 21 (1) years, mass: 61.8 (6.4) kg, and height: 166 (5) cm]. Volunteers were accepted if they had no history of lower extremity injury requiring surgical repair, and had not suffered a knee injury within the previous 6 months. Recreationally active was defined as being physically active in running and cutting activities (i.e. soccer, volleyball, tennis, basketball, etc.) at least 3 times per week for a minimum of 30 min. Additionally, participants were required to be pain-free in the lower extremity on testing days	Influence of movement anticipation on ACL loading	(i) Limitations: (1) Optimization theory was not used to predict muscle coordination during sidestep cutting. (2) Although many model parameters such as muscle FOM, segment masses, and lengths were participant-specific estimates, others such as posterior tibial slope was an average of cadaveric data.

Table C.5.　Characteristics of included studies: Case control study form.

Study	Country	Setting/context	Participant characteristics	Group A description and sample	Group B description and sample	Exposures/variables measured	Description of main results
Lin, C-Y, Shau, Y-W, Wang, C-L and Kang, J-H (2015)	Taiwan	(i) To investigate how the viscoelastic properties of the ankle ligament complex can be used to quantitatively assess inversion ankle sprains (IAS). (ii) To investigate the usefulness of the stretched exponential function to analyze the relaxation behavior of the ankle ligament complex	Two groups of participants with no significant difference in age or gender	(1) Injured group with IAS: 10 men and five women who experienced unilateral IAS within 1 year of the study	(2) Control group: 10 men and five women without any ankle injury on either of their ankles during the 2 years prior to the study	Statistical analysis was performed to determine differences in the viscoelastic properties and relaxation behavior of the injured and control groups	(i) This study proves that one can use a mathematical model to analyze the relaxation behavior of ligaments, specifically the ankle ligament complex, using an instrumented anterior drawer test that monitors force. (ii) Sprained and unsprained ankles have vastly different relaxation behaviors and viscoelastic properties: (1) Sprained ankles exhibit significantly less viscous response than uninjured ankles. (iii) Therefore, inversion ankle sprains cause significant changes to the viscoelastic properties of the ankle.

CHAPTER 6

Assessment of Gait Balance Control Using Inertial Measurement Units — A Narrative Review[a]

Yu-Pin Liang[*] and Li-Shan Chou[†]

Department of Kinesiology, Iowa State University,
235 Forker Building, 534 Wallace Road, Ames, IA 50011, USA
[*]yupinl@iastate.edu
[†]chou@iastate.edu

This narrative review examines the use of inertial measurement units (IMUs) for assessing gait balance control. Impaired gait balance control is associated with an increased risk of falls and reduced mobility, particularly in older adults. Traditional methods of assessing gait balance control, such as clinical balance assessments and camera-based motion analysis, have limitations in terms of reliability, cost, and practicality. Wearable sensor technology, including IMUs, offers a more accessible and cost-effective alternative for assessing gait and balance performance in real-world settings. IMUs, equipped with tri-axial accelerometers, gyroscopes, and magnetometers, can directly measure body movement and provide quantifiable data. This review explores the advantages and limitations of using IMUs for assessing gait balance control, including the measurement of anticipatory postural adjustments (APAs) for gait initiation, spatiotemporal gait parameters, center of mass (COM) motion during walking, and data-driven machine learning models. IMUs have shown promise in quantifying APAs, estimating gait spatiotemporal parameters, assessing COM motion, and using machine learning algorithms to classify and predict balance-related outcomes. However, further research is needed to establish standardized protocols, validate IMU-based measurements, and determine the specific IMU parameters that correlate with balance control ability. Overall, IMUs have the potential to be a valuable tool for assessing gait balance control, monitoring changes over time, and tracking interventions to improve balance control in both clinical and research settings.

Keywords: Inertial measurement units (IMU); gait; balance control; falls; anticipatory posture adjustment (APA); whole-body center of mass (COM); artificial neural networks (ANN).

[†]Corresponding author.
[a]This article was previously published in *World Scientific Annual Review of Biomechanics*. Vol: 1, (2023) 2330006 (10 pages).

1. Introduction

Gait balance control refers to the ability to maintain postural stability and controlled movement during walking (Winter, 2009). Impaired gait balance control has been associated with an increased risk of falls and reduced mobility in various populations. For instance, individuals with neurological conditions, such as Parkinson's disease, multiple sclerosis, or stroke, may experience gait disturbances and impaired balance control (Khanmohammadi *et al.*, 2018). However, the risk of falls and injuries associated with impaired gait balance control is exceptionally high in the elderly population. In the United States, falls are a major public health concern with millions of older adults falling each year (Bergen *et al.*, 2016; Moreland *et al.*, 2020). In 2020, over 36,000 fatalities occurred as a result of falls, making them the primary cause of unintentional injury-related deaths among older adults (Centers for Disease Control and Prevention, 2020). Falls can result in severe injuries, including hip fractures or traumatic brain injuries (TBIs), and can significantly impact an individual's quality of life and pose significant personal and social-economic burdens (Sterling *et al.*, 2001; Florence *et al.*, 2018). Thus, the ability to assess and improve gait balance control is essential for reducing the risk of falls and promoting healthy aging.

Falls are caused by a range of factors, including both extrinsic environmental factors and intrinsic individual factors (Berg *et al.*, 1997). Cognitive function, as well as the condition of musculoskeletal and neurological systems, play critical roles in gait balance and posture control, and these functions can be compromised by age-related degeneration or diseases, such as Alzheimer's or Parkinson's disease (Savica *et al.*, 2017; Verghese *et al.*, 2002). Balance control during walking involves regulating the position of the whole-body center of mass (COM) relative to the base of support in order to maintain stability (Shumway-Cook and Woollacott, 2007). Poor gait balance control has been identified as a leading risk factor for falls (Salzman, 2010), and altered COM motion during walking may indicate gait imbalance (Howell *et al.*, 2013). In addition to reducing the risk of falls and injuries, balance control is also essential for athletes, as it can help improve their return-to-play performance and prevent sports-related injuries (Paillard, 2017).

Two main approaches for assessing balance control ability are performance-oriented clinical assessment and biomechanical analysis of body movement. Most clinical balance assessments focus on functional balance evaluation and individual movement behavior when dealing with environmental balance disturbances and translate them into quantifiable ratings. Common clinical balance assessments include the modified Berg Balance Scale (mBBS), Timed Up and Go

(TUG) test in the STEADI Algorithm, and Tinetti Balance and Gait Assessment, which focus on evaluating dynamic balance control and identifying individuals at higher risk of falling (Blum and Korner-Bitensky, 2008; Ng and Hui-Chan, 2005; Tinetti *et al.*, 1986). In contrast, biomechanical analysis estimates kinetic and kinematic parameters during movement to objectively quantify balance control. For example, the spatiotemporal gait variables and the COM kinematics have been shown to detect balance impairments and predict fall risk (Horak, 2006). Both performance-oriented assessment and biomechanical measurements are essential tools for assessing balance control ability, and each approach has advantages and limitations.

Functional balance tests, such as the Tinetti Balance and Gait Assessment and the STEADI Algorithm from CDC, are widely used to evaluate balance control ability in clinical settings. However, these tests rely heavily on the examiner's experience and could result in inconsistent inter- and intra-rater reliability (Rockwood *et al.*, 2000). Furthermore, such overall performance ratings or measures might not provide information on underlying mechanisms leading to gait imbalance. On the other hand, the laboratory-based biomechanical movement analysis, employing camera-based motion capture systems and force platforms, could provide comprehensive kinematic and kinetic data to objectively quantify gait balance performance and biomechanical causes of gait imbalance (Winter, 2009). However, such comprehensive biomechanical assessments are not always feasible in real-world or clinical settings due to its high equipment costs and extensive expertise required for data acquisition and analysis. As a result, more straightforward and cost-effective methods for assessing gait balance control are being developed to improve the clinical utility of balance assessments.

Wearable sensor technology has made significant strides in recent years, offering a more practical and convenient means of assessing an individual's mobility without environmental limitations. These devices are equipped with multiple sensors, including tri-axial accelerometers, gyroscopes, and magnetometers, and, which are collectively known as inertial measurement units (IMUs). IMUs enable researchers to directly measure body movement and collect quantifiable data in various daily activities. With their time-efficient and user-friendly features, wearable sensors have become a popular alternative for estimating gait and balance performance (O'Sullivan *et al.*, 2009; Pitt and Chou, 2019). Compared to traditional methods that rely on camera-based motion capture systems in a laboratory setting, wearable sensors are less costly and easy to operate and could be accessible to real-world environments.

This review was, therefore, aimed to examine the current literature on the advanced assessment of gait and balance control, with a specific focus on the use of IMUs. The review explored the advantages and limitations of using wearable sensors in clinical and research settings. Additionally, the review discussed the potential of wearable sensors for identifying individuals at risk for falls, monitoring changes in gait and balance over time, and assessing the effectiveness of interventions to improve balance control. Ultimately, this review would provide a comprehensive overview of the current state of wearable sensor technology for gait and balance assessment and highlight its potential for future clinical and research applications.

2. Methods

A search was conducted in the PubMed database using the terms "gait and balance control" and ("IMU" or "inertial" or "wearable sensor") in all search fields, with a filter for full-text articles published from 2011 to 2022. This initial search yielded a total of 99 articles. Articles were excluded if (1) gait-related activities were not included in the experimental protocols, (2) there was no outcome measurement to evaluate gait balance performance, or (3) it was a review paper. Thus, a total of 25 articles were included in this review.

Human walking is categorized into three phases, including gait initiation, steady-state walking, and gait termination (Winter, 2009). Most studies that used IMUs to examine balance control were during steady-state walking using derived gait spatiotemporal parameters or kinematic data obtained from an IMU attached to the fifth lumbar vertebra, a proxy location for the whole-body COM. There is an increasing number of studies employing artificial neural network algorithms or similar machine learning approaches to map IMU data with desired outcome variables. IMU's feasibility to collect body movement data from functional activities in real-world settings provides a significant amount of valuable human movement data for training of machine learning models. In the following session, we discussed the use of IMU for assessing balance control during walking in three parts: (1) the anticipatory postural adjustments (APAs) for gait initiation, (2) steady-state walking, and (3) data-driven machine learning model.

3. Discussion

3.1. *APA for gait initiation*

Anticipatory posture adjustment is required for balance maintenance and gait initiation and is an important indicator of an individual's balance control ability (Lepers and Brenière, 1995). Typically, APA is examined using force platforms to trace the center of pressure trajectory during gait initiation. Recent studies have shown that IMU can also be used to quantify APAs in various populations (Bonora *et al.*, 2017a,b; Lencioni *et al.*, 2022; Martinez-Mendez *et al.*, 2011). For instance, similar amplitudes and durations of APAs could be measured when using IMU sensors attached to the lower back with one footswitch and the stabilometer (Martinez-Mendez *et al.*, 2011). In addition, significant correlations have been found between temporal parameters extracted from wearable sensors and force platforms, as well as between the mediolateral trunk acceleration and COP displacement, which support the validity of using IMU to evaluate APAs prior to both gait initiation and stair ascending in patients with Parkinson's disease (Bonora *et al.*, 2015, 2017b). IMU data also provided important insights on changes in APA strategy under different environmental settings in patients with spinal cord injuries (Fantozzi *et al.*, 2022). Furthermore, IMU data were reported to detect and distinguish APAs and gait events in Parkinson's gait, which could enhance our understanding of underlying mechanisms contributing to gait impairments (Lencioni *et al.*, 2022). Finally, APA magnitudes detected with IMU data were reported to be associated ventricle volume in healthy controls, but not in individuals with Parkinson's disease (Ragothaman *et al.*, 2022).

3.2. *Steady-state walking*

3.2.1. *Gait spatiotemporal parameters*

Gait performance is a sensitive indicator of balance control and mobility, and, therefore, a quantitative gait assessment could be critical to diagnoses of gait disorders or balance impairment. IMUs attached to shoes or upper extremities have shown promising results in estimating these parameters in various populations. Increased stride time variability has been linked to early dementia, which can lead to a high risk of falls (Montero-Odasso *et al.*, 2012). IMU data have been shown to be sensitive to changes in gait parameters due to the progression of Parkinson's disease (Buckley *et al.*, 2019; Schlachetzki *et al.*, 2017). In fact, there is excellent agreement between GAITRite measures and estimates from wearable sensor data for most temporal gait measures, such as stance time, step time, and gait velocity, as well as for step count in different age groups (O'Brien *et al.*, 2019).

IMUs have also been applied in fall prevention studies to monitor gait changes in patients with diabetes, neurodegenerative disorders, or multiple sclerosis (Brognara *et al.*, 2021; Das *et al.*, 2022; Huang *et al.*, 2022). It was reported, based on the data collected from community-dwelling older adults, that IMUs provided reliable spatiotemporal measures with data from three consecutive gait cycles and good reliability for most parameters describing gait variability and asymmetry from six gait cycles (Motti Ader *et al.*, 2021).

IMU data could be used to estimate gait acceleration intensity, variability, and stability. In a study comparing young and old females, trunk mediolateral acceleration amplitude, maximum vertical acceleration, amplitude, and gait variability were significantly larger in older females (Zhang *et al.*, 2021). Moreover, older females showed lower stability in trunk mediolateral acceleration and vertical angular velocity, indicating a higher fall risk.

3.2.2. *COM motion during walking*

The motion of the whole-body COM reflects the overall mechanical effect on an individual and has been frequently assessed in the study of human locomotion, especially when examining balance control during standing or walking (Hof, 2008; Pai and Patton, 1997; Winter, 1995). Altered COM motion has been reported in individuals with gait dysfunction, and many COM-related kinematic markers have been identified to sensitively detect gait imbalance (Hahn and Chou, 2004; Kaya *et al.*, 1998).

Age-related reductions in the sagittal plane COM motion were reported during walking and obstacle crossing (Hahn and Chou, 2004). Increased frontal plane COM displacement and peak velocity during walking were reported in older fallers (Lee and Chou, 2006) and in concussed young adults during dual-task walking (Howell *et al.*, 2013). Moreover, COM accelerations have been reported to better differentiate between individuals with and without functional limitations (Fujimoto and Chou, 2012, 2014) and to identify individuals with balance control deficits during daily activities.

Recent studies have utilized a single accelerometer placed over the fifth lumbar vertebrae (L5) as a proxy for the whole-body COM to examine gait acceleration control and concluded that such acceleration data were reliable, clinically practical, and could be sensitive to detect gait imbalance (Howell *et al.*, 2015; Pitt and Chou, 2019). In longitudinal studies tracking recovery after concussion, the root mean square of mediolateral sway during walking derived from IMU data was greater in individuals with concussion (Parrington *et al.*, 2019). Therefore, using IMUs to estimate COM motion and assess gait balance control in older adults and various patient populations is highly feasible.

3.3. *IMU data-driven machine learning models*

Wearable devices greatly enhance our ability to collect body movement data from functional activities and provide real-world data that can be used as inputs for machine learning models to classify categorical outcome measurements or predict regression variables. For example, using data from a single foot-worn sensor during walking and a long short-term memory model, the center of pressure position could be accurately predicted (Podobnik *et al.*, 2020; Wu *et al.*, 2020). IMU data during walking have been used to classify individuals with balance impairments using various machine learning algorithms, including the back propagation artificial neural network (Di Lazzaro *et al.*, 2020), support vector machine (Nguyen *et al.*, 2019a), *k*-nearest neighbors (Nukala *et al.*, 2016), and binary decision trees (Nguyen *et al.*, 2019b). Furthermore, machine learning-based random forest methods have demonstrated a high accuracy (99.83%) in distinguishing compensatory balance response events from normal walking (Nouredanesh and Tung, 2019).

In the context of fall risk assessment in patients with Parkinson's disease, a deep neural network model was employed to estimate individual segments' contributions to angular momentum with IMU data (Pickle *et al.*, 2019). Gait features extracted from IMU data during the TUG test have been shown to classify individuals with Parkinson's disease or essential tremor (Moon *et al.*, 2020), while data from two IMUs placed on each shin during the same test can predict freezing gait before it occurs in patients with Parkinson's disease (Borzì *et al.*, 2021). It is important to carefully select and weigh the features extracted from IMU data before training a machine learning model to predict different balance outcome measurements (Ko *et al.*, 2022). Overall, these studies highlight the potential of IMU data-driven machine learning models to accurately classify and predict balance-related outcomes, which would provide insights into gait and balance control and improve the clinical decision-making.

4. Conclusion

In conclusion, IMUs could be a promising tool for assessing gait balance control in real-world settings, offering a cost-effective and user-friendly alternative to traditional laboratory-based methods. However, standardized protocols and computational algorithms may need to be developed and validated to ensure the reliability and validity of IMU-based measurements. More research is needed to establish the relationship between specific IMU measurements or parameters and balance control ability. Overall, the findings from this review suggest that IMUs could be an accessible and effective technology to quantify and monitor critical body movement during activities of daily living and provide objective data to inform the development of targeted interventions to improve gait balance control.

References

Berg, WP, Alessio, HM, Mills, EM and Tong, C (1997) Circumstances and consequences of falls in independent community-dwelling older adults, *Age Ageing* **26**(4), 261–268, doi:10.1093/ageing/26.4.261.

Bergen, G, Stevens, MR and Burns, ER (2016) Falls and fall injuries among adults aged ≥65 years — United States, 2014, *Morb. Mortal. Wkly. Rep.* **65**(37), 993–998, doi:10.15585/mmwr.mm6537a2.

Blum, L and Korner-Bitensky, N (2008) Usefulness of the Berg Balance Scale in stroke rehabilitation: A systematic review, *Phys. Ther.* **88**(5), 559–566, doi:10.2522/ptj.20070205.

Bonora, G, Carpinella, I, Cattaneo, D, Chiari, L and Ferrarin, M (2015) A new instrumented method for the evaluation of gait initiation and step climbing based on inertial sensors: A pilot application in Parkinson's disease, *J. NeuroEng. Rehabil.* **12**, 45, doi:10.1186/s12984-015-0038-0.

Bonora, G, Mancini, M, Carpinella, I, Chiari, L, Ferrarin, M, Nutt, JG and Horak, FB (2017a) Investigation of anticipatory postural adjustments during one-leg stance using inertial sensors: Evidence from subjects with Parkinsonism, *Front. Neurol.* **8**, 361, doi:10.3389/fneur.2017.00361.

Bonora, G, Mancini, M, Carpinella, I, Chiari, L, Horak, FB and Ferrarin, M (2017b) Gait initiation is impaired in subjects with Parkinson's disease in the OFF state: Evidence from the analysis of the anticipatory postural adjustments through wearable inertial sensors, *Gait Posture* **51**, 218–221, doi:10.1016/j.gaitpost.2016.10.017.

Borzì, L, Mazzetta, I, Zampogna, A, Suppa, A, Olmo, G and Irrera, F (2021) Prediction of freezing of gait in Parkinson's disease using wearables and machine learning, *Sensors (Basel)* **21**(2), 614, doi:10.3390/s21020614.

Brognara, L, Mazzotti, A, Di Martino, A, Faldini, C and Cauli, O (2021) Wearable sensor for assessing gait and postural alterations in patients with diabetes: A scoping review, *Medicina (Kaunas)* **57**(11), 1145, doi:10.3390/medicina57111145.

Buckley, C, Galna, B, Rochester, L and Mazzà, C (2019) Upper body accelerations as a biomarker of gait impairment in the early stages of Parkinson's disease, *Gait Posture* **71**, 289–295, doi:10.1016/j.gaitpost.2018.06.166.

Centers for Disease Control and Prevention (2020) Web-based injury statistics query and reporting system (WISQARS), National Center for Injury Prevention and Control, URL https://www.cdc.gov/injury/wisqars/ (retrieved 10 July 2023).

Das, R, Paul, S, Mourya, GK, Kumar, N and Hussain, M (2022) Recent trends and practices toward assessment and rehabilitation of neurodegenerative disorders: Insights from human gait, *Front. Neurosci.* **16**, 859298, doi:10.3389/fnins.2022.859298.

Di Lazzaro, G, Ricci, M, Al-Wardat, M, Schirinzi, T, Scalise, S, Giannini, F, Mercuri, N, Saggio, G and Pisani, A (2020) Technology-based objective measures detect subclinical axial signs in untreated, *de novo* Parkinson's disease, *J. Parkinson's Dis.* **10**(1), 113–122, doi:10.3233/jpd-191758.

Fantozzi, S, Borra, D, Cortesi, M, Ferrari, A, Ciacci, S, Chiari, L and Baroncini, I (2022) Aquatic therapy after incomplete spinal cord injury: Gait initiation analysis using inertial sensors, *Int. J. Environ. Res. Public Health* **19**(18), 11568, doi:10.3390/ijerph191811568.

Florence, CS, Bergen, G, Atherly, A, Burns, E, Stevens, J and Drake, C (2018) Medical costs of fatal and nonfatal falls in older adults, *J. Am. Geriatr. Soc.* **66**(4), 693–698, doi:10.1111/jgs.15304.

Fujimoto, M and Chou, LS (2012) Dynamic balance control during sit-to-stand movement: An examination with the center of mass acceleration, *J. Biomech.* **45**(3), 543–548, doi:10.1016/j.jbiomech.2011.11.037.

Fujimoto, M and Chou, LS (2014) Region of stability derived by center of mass acceleration better identifies individuals with difficulty in sit-to-stand movement, *Ann. Biomed. Eng.* **42**(4), 733–741, doi:10.1007/s10439-013-0945-9.

Hahn, ME and Chou, LS (2004) Age-related reduction in sagittal plane center of mass motion during obstacle crossing, *J. Biomech.* **37**(6), 837–844, doi:10.1016/j.jbiomech.2003.11.010.

Hof, AL (2008) The "extrapolated center of mass" concept suggests a simple control of balance in walking, *Hum. Mov. Sci.* **27**(1), 112–125, doi:10.1016/j.humov.2007.08.003.

Horak, FB (2006) Postural orientation and equilibrium: What do we need to know about neural control of balance to prevent falls? *Age Ageing* **35**(Suppl. 2), ii7–ii11, doi:10.1093/ageing/afl077.

Howell, DR, Osternig, LR and Chou, LS (2013) Dual-task effect on gait balance control in adolescents with concussion, *Arch. Phys. Med. Rehabil.* **94**(8), 1513–1520, doi:10.1016/j.apmr.2013.04.015.

Howell, D, Osternig, L and Chou, LS (2015) Monitoring recovery of gait balance control following concussion using an accelerometer, *J. Biomech.* **48**(12), 3364–3368, doi:10.1016/j.jbiomech.2015.06.014.

Huang, SC, Guerrieri, S, Dalla Costa, G, Pisa, M, Leccabue, G, Gregoris, L, Comi, G and Leocani, L (2022) Intensive neurorehabilitation and gait improvement in progressive multiple sclerosis: Clinical, kinematic and electromyographic analysis, *Brain Sci.* **12**(2), 258, doi:10.3390/brainsci12020258.

Kaya, BK, Krebs, DE and Riley, PO (1998) Dynamic stability in elders: Momentum control in locomotor ADL, *J. Gerontol. A Biol. Sci. Med. Sci.* **53**(2), M126–M134, doi:10.1093/gerona/53a.2.m126.

Ko, JB, Hong, JS, Shin, YS and Kim, KB (2022) Machine learning-based predicted age of the elderly on the instrumented timed up and go test and six-minute walk test, *Sensors (Basel)* **22**(16), 5957, doi:10.3390/s22165957.

Lee, HJ and Chou, LS (2006) Detection of gait instability using the center of mass and center of pressure inclination angles, *Arch. Phys. Med. Rehabil.* **87**(4), 569–575, doi:10.1016/j.apmr.2005.11.033.

Lencioni, T, Meloni, M, Bowman, T, Marzegan, A, Caronni, A, Carpinella, I, Castagna, A, Gower, V, Ferrarin, M and Pelosin, E (2022) Events detection of anticipatory postural adjustments through a wearable accelerometer sensor is comparable to that measured by the force platform in subjects with Parkinson's disease, *Sensors (Basel)* **22**(7), 2668, doi:10.3390/s22072668.

Lepers, R and Brenière, Y (1995) The role of anticipatory postural adjustments and gravity in gait initiation, *Exp. Brain Res.* **107**(1), 118–124, doi:10.1007/bf00228023.

Martinez-Mendez, R, Sekine, M and Tamura, T (2011) Detection of anticipatory postural adjustments prior to gait initiation using inertial wearable sensors, *J. Neuroeng. Rehabil.* **8**, 17, doi:10.1186/1743-0003-8-17.

Montero-Odasso, M, Verghese, J, Beauchet, O and Hausdorff, JM (2012) Gait and cognition: A complementary approach to understanding brain function and the risk of falling, *J. Am. Geriatr. Soc.* **60**(11), 2127–2136, doi:10.1111/j.1532-5415.2012.04209.x.

Moon, S, Song, HJ, Sharma, VD, Lyons, KE, Pahwa, R, Akinwuntan, AE and Devos, H (2020) Classification of Parkinson's disease and essential tremor based on balance and gait characteristics from wearable motion sensors via machine learning techniques: A data-driven approach, *J. Neuroeng. Rehabil.* **17**(1), 125, doi:10.1186/s12984-020-00756-5.

Moreland, B, Kakara, R and Henry, A (2020) Trends in nonfatal falls and fall-related injuries among adults aged ≥65 years — United States, 2012–2018, *Morb. Mortal. Wkly. Rep.* **69**(27), 875–881, doi:10.15585/mmwr.mm6927a5.

Motti Ader, LG, Greene, BR, McManus, K and Caulfield, B (2021) Reliability of inertial sensor based spatiotemporal gait parameters for short walking bouts in community dwelling older adults, *Gait Posture* **85**, 1–6, doi:10.1016/j.gaitpost.2021.01.010.

Ng, SS and Hui-Chan, CW (2005) The timed up & go test: Its reliability and association with lower-limb impairments and locomotor capacities in people with chronic stroke, *Arch. Phys. Med. Rehabil.* **86**(8), 1641–1647, doi:10.1016/j.apmr.2005.01.011.

Nguyen, A, Roth, N, Ghassemi, NH, Hannink, J, Seel, T, Klucken, J, Gassner, H and Eskofier, BM (2019a) Development and clinical validation of inertial sensor-based gait-clustering methods in Parkinson's disease, *J. Neuroeng. Rehabil.* **16**(1), 77, doi:10.1186/s12984-019-0548-2.

Nguyen, TQ, Young, JH, Rodriguez, A, Zupancic, S and Lie, DYC (2019b) Differentiation of patients with balance insufficiency (vestibular hypofunction) versus normal subjects using a low-cost small wireless wearable gait sensor, *Biosensors (Basel)* **9**(1), 29, doi:10.3390/bios9010029.

Nouredanesh, M and Tung, J (2019) IMU, sEMG, or their cross-correlation and temporal similarities: Which signal features detect lateral compensatory balance reactions more accurately? *Comput. Methods Programs Biomed.* **182**, 105003, doi:10.1016/j.cmpb.2019.105003.

Nukala, BT, Nakano, T, Rodriguez, A, Tsay, J, Lopez, J, Nguyen, TQ, Zupancic, S and Lie, DY (2016) Real-time classification of patients with balance disorders vs. normal subjects using a low-cost small wireless wearable gait sensor, *Biosensors (Basel)* **6**(4), 58, doi:10.3390/bios6040058.

O'Brien, MK, Hidalgo-Araya, MD, Mummidisetty, CK, Vallery, H, Ghaffari, R, Rogers, JA, Lieber, R and Jayaraman, A (2019) Augmenting clinical outcome measures of gait and balance with a single inertial sensor in age-ranged healthy adults, *Sensors (Basel)* **19**(20), 4537, doi:10.3390/s19204537.

O'Sullivan, M, Blake, C, Cunningham, C, Boyle, G and Finucane, C (2009) Correlation of accelerometry with clinical balance tests in older fallers and non-fallers, *Age Ageing* **38**(3), 308–313, doi:10.1093/ageing/afp009.

Pai, YC and Patton, J (1997) Center of mass velocity-position predictions for balance control, *J. Biomech.* **30**(4), 347–354, doi:10.1016/s0021-9290(96)00165-0.

Parrington, L, Fino, PC, Swanson, CW, Murchison, CF, Chesnutt, J and King, LA (2019) Longitudinal assessment of balance and gait after concussion and return to play in collegiate athletes, *J. Athl. Train.* **54**(4), 429–438, doi:10.4085/1062-6050-46-18.

Pickle, NT, Shearin, SM and Fey, NP (2019) Dynamic neural network approach to targeted balance assessment of individuals with and without neurological disease during non-steady-state locomotion, *J. Neuroeng. Rehabil.* **16**(1), 88, doi:10.1186/s12984-019-0550-8.

Pitt, W and Chou, LS (2019) Reliability and practical clinical application of an accelerometer-based dual-task gait balance control assessment, *Gait Posture* **71**, 279–283, doi:10.1016/j.gaitpost.2019.05.014.

Podobnik, J, Kraljić, D, Zadravec, M and Munih, M (2020) Centre of pressure estimation during walking using only inertial-measurement units and end-to-end statistical modelling, *Sensors (Basel)* **20**(21), 6136, doi:10.3390/s20216136.

Ragothaman, A, Mancini, M, Nutt, JG, Fair, DA, Miranda-Dominguez, O and Horak, FB (2022) Resting state functional networks predict different aspects of postural control in Parkinson's disease, *Gait Posture* **97**, 122–129, doi:10.1016/j.gaitpost.2022.07.003.

Rockwood, K, Awalt, E, Carver, D and MacKnight, C (2000) Feasibility and measurement properties of the functional reach and the timed up and go tests in the Canadian study of health and aging, *J. Gerontol. A Biol. Sci. Med. Sci.* **55**(2), M70–M73, doi:10.1093/gerona/55.2.m70.

Salzman, B (2010) Gait and balance disorders in older adults, *Am. Fam. Physician* **82**(1), 61–68.

Savica, R, Wennberg, AM, Hagen, C, Edwards, K, Roberts, RO, Hollman, JH, Knopman, DS, Boeve, BF, Machulda, MM, Petersen, RC and Mielke, MM (2017) Comparison of gait parameters for predicting cognitive decline: The Mayo Clinic Study of Aging, *J. Alzheimer's Dis.* **55**(2), 559–567, doi:10.3233/jad-160697.

Schlachetzki, JCM, Barth, J, Marxreiter, F, Gossler, J, Kohl, Z, Reinfelder, S, Gassner, H, Aminian, K, Eskofier, BM, Winkler, J and Klucken, J (2017) Wearable sensors objectively measure gait parameters in Parkinson's disease, *PLoS One* **12**(10), e0183989, doi:10.1371/journal.pone.0183989.

Shumway-Cook, A and Woollacott, MH (2007) *Motor Control: Translating Research into Clinical Practice* (Lippincott Williams & Wilkins).

Sterling, DA, O'Connor, JA and Bonadies, J (2001) Geriatric falls: Injury severity is high and disproportionate to mechanism, *J. Trauma* **50**(1), 116–119, doi:10.1097/00005373-200101000-00021.

Tinetti, ME, Williams, TF and Mayewski, R (1986) Fall risk index for elderly patients based on number of chronic disabilities, *Am. J. Med.* **80**(3), 429–434, doi:10.1016/0002-9343(86)90717-5.

Verghese, J, Lipton, RB, Hall, CB, Kuslansky, G, Katz, MJ and Buschke, H (2002) Abnormality of gait as a predictor of non-Alzheimer's dementia, *N. Engl. J. Med.* **347**(22), 1761–1768, doi:10.1056/NEJMoa020441.

Winter, DA (1995) Human balance and posture control during standing and walking, *Gait Posture* **3**(4), 193–214, doi:10.1016/0966-6362(96)82849-9.

Winter, DA (2009). *Biomechanics and Motor Control of Human Movement* (Wiley).

Wu, CC, Chen, YJ, Hsu, CS, Wen, YT and Lee, YJ (2020) Multiple inertial measurement unit combination and location for center of pressure prediction in gait, *Front. Bioeng. Biotechnol.* **8**, 566474, doi:10.3389/fbioe.2020.566474.

Zhang, Y, Zhou, X, Pijnappels, M and Bruijn, SM (2021) Differences in gait stability and acceleration characteristics between healthy young and older females, *Front. Rehabil. Sci.* **2**, 763309, doi:10.3389/fresc.2021.763309.

www.ingramcontent.com/pod-product-compliance
Lightning Source LLC
Chambersburg PA
CBHW050752150726
48196CB00004B/437